KAMA SUTRA SEX POSITIONS:

Transform your Sexual Life and Relationship with Tantric Sex.

Amplify Pleasure and Longevity Using Oral Sex to Deepen Emotional and Physical Intimacy and Reach Multiple Orgasms.

Abigail Eros

Table of Contents

Introduction

Kama Sutra is an ancient Indian text on the sexual behavior of humans, written by Malanga Vatsyayana, an Indian scholar. It contains practical advice about sexual intercourse and other things related to relationships, finding the girl, and keeping her (them).

Kama means sexual pleasure, while Sutra means a line or a thread that holds things together.

The "Discipline of Kama" came from Nandi, the sacred bull, which was Shiva's doorkeeper, who was moved to sacred words upon overhearing the God and his wife, Parvati, making love. His words were recorded to benefit all of mankind.

The purpose of the Kama Sutra, first and foremost, is to acquire knowledge. In terms of sexual union, Kama Sutra aims to stimulate each partner's desires. Partners are also taught of ideal sexual intercourse positions that can give the ultimate pleasure and orgasm.

It even teaches gestures and actions besides the actual sexual intercourse. Everything comes together for every couple's ultimate sexual experience.

A man will also learn how to "get" the girl. Kama Sutra also teaches readers about the different forms of marriage. However, it is not just about having a partner; Kama Sutra also gives insights on how a person can manage to live alone.

Tantra is a practical application of utilizing biochemical transformations in the body in order to facilitate increased states of awareness. Tantric principles say that sex has three purposes:

- Pleasure.

- Liberation—Couples looking for liberation will eschew frictional orgasm in order to reach a higher form of ecstasy.

- Procreation.

Taoism (also known as Daoism) refers to many different yet related philosophical and religious traditions. Its influences came from the Eastern Asia area. Taoism has been in existence for over two millennia. The Western cultures have been adapting Taoism principles since the start of the 19th century.

The term tao literally means way or path.

Sexuality According to Taoism

Do not view your body as a dangerous source of temptation. It is a positive asset.

The body is a vital component of romantic love. Taoism, however, reiterates that people need to practice self-control and moderation.

One's complete abstinence from sex contains the same "dangers" to having excessive sexual indulgence.

The vitality of men in sex is often portrayed as something limited. On the other hand, women's sexual energy is considered to be boundless.

The men are taught to control ejaculation in order to preserve their vital energy in sex, but women are encouraged to achieve orgasmic pleasure without limitations.

Practitioners believe that a man can nourish his own vital energy by bringing his woman to pure orgasmic pleasure, thus allowing her to "activate" her own sexual vitality so that it is attuned with his man.

Couples have a lot to learn from these three principles when it comes to sex and achieving ultimate sexual pleasures. As you continue to read, you'll find 11 sex positions that are guaranteed to ignite you and your partner's sexual passion and desire for each other.

Remember that great sex contributes to a great relationship between two people.

Kama Sutra is more popular than Tantric Sex. Kama Sutra is more about teaching couples how to have the most amazing sex ever as it teaches different techniques and positions on how to enjoy sex. The Kama Sutra also includes different tips on how to reach ultimate orgasmic sex each time intercourse happens.

Many people do not know about Tantra or Tantric Sex; this will give you an idea of what it is all about and how it is different or similar to the Kama Sutra.

Tantra embraces all the natural energies that the body produces and how they are connected to the universal energy. Tantric Sex means being one with your partner and the very cosmos or universe itself.

The word "Tantra" means weave (thread), so when you say Tantric Sex, it is like weaving together the bodies of two separate individuals to become and move as one. There is interdependence and continuity of interaction between bodies until a spiritual and divine connection is achieved.

The Tantra philosophy was founded on the unity and interaction of the universe with living things. The human body cannot exist alone because it is a part of "The One" and connected with the entire universe.

The human body is a microcosm of the universe, meaning everything that exists in the universe also exists in the body. The real path of enlightenment is through the realization and establishment of your connection to the dynamic unit of the universe and the energy of reality.

Through Tantric Sex and the intimate connection of the body and the universe, you can achieve the most divine experience. Tantric Sex is used in order to enhance energies, consciousness, and your connection to the universe as a whole in order to find healing, peace, joy, happiness, and personal growth.

A lot of ideas of the Tantric philosophy are based on other branches of philosophical principles and traditions. They include Thales and Heraclitus from the Greeks, Zeno and Marcus Aurelius from Stoicism, and Taoism. Even Albert Einstein was able to prove the interconnection and unity of all things in the universe. The belief that all is one and interconnected does have a metaphysical foundation and is not merely fabricated on false beliefs and theories.

Chapter 1. Tantric Sex

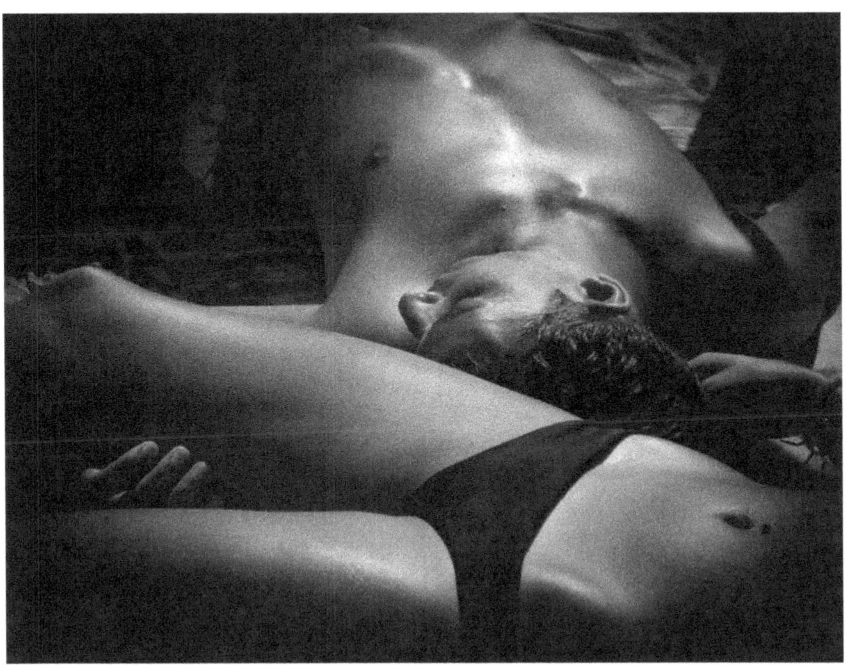

What Is Tantric Sex?

Tantric Sex is derived from something called the Tantra, which is a very old spiritual practice. For our purposes, we will be primarily looking at how the Tantra practice relates to sex and not at the other facets of this type of spirituality, though they are inextricably linked. In the way that Tantra has become related to sex, it can be viewed as a sort of new-age or Neo-Tantra. This is a modern take on Tantra that links it to sex and sex positions that we hear about most often today in the Western World.

Tantric Sex or Neotantra is essentially spiritual sex. It takes the old beliefs and teachings of Tantra and brings them into our modern relationships and sex lives in order to help us better connect in our romantic relationships and to be one with our bodies and sensations. This type of sex is great for couples and long-term relationships. One of the main focuses of Tantric Sex is a mutual exchange of energy between partners. Another focus is getting in touch with the sensations and feelings of your body. It is also about removing distractions and being mindful in order to have more intense, longer-lasting, full-body orgasms, and being mindful means to bring your consciousness and awareness to the present moment. It is the state of being fully present in your body, your actions, and thoughts, and noticing them as they change. Being in this state allows you to feel the physical sensations within your body and removes the distraction of a mind full of running thoughts.

The Science Behind Tantric Sex

In Tantric Sex, everything comes down to the belief that women are generally taught to always focus on the needs of others and on taking care of others, as well as to place more importance on the pleasure of others than on themselves. It is believed that women are so disconnected from their feelings and sensations that they must begin a practice of mindfulness in order to reconnect with their feelings and sensations.

Tantric Theory states that women have a more difficult time than men when it comes to reaching orgasm. Specifically, it states that women are quite preoccupied with the duties of the household, including the children and their needs, the household and its needs, their work, their friends, and anything and anyone else in their lives. They are also preoccupied with subtle distractions such as noises or the temperature, demonstrating that they are always on high alert in an attempt to ensure everything is running smoothly and that nobody is uncomfortable in any way. This is similar to what we discussed when we looked at how to get in the right mindset for sex in terms of removing distractions and prioritizing foreplay.

In short, Tantric Theory is of the belief that women are raised to focus on the pleasure and wellbeing of others and are, as a result, out of touch completely with their own bodies, their own pleasure, and their own desires (these desires can be both of a sexual nature and otherwise, but here, we will focus on the sexual desires). Because of this, when it comes to sex, women tend to be unable to put aside their focus on others and turn that focus inward to themselves. When in a long-term relationship, they will be so invested in the pleasure of their partner that they will not focus on their own. Even in a casual sexual encounter, the woman will be focused on ensuring that she is giving the man a good time at the expense of her own pleasure.

To further its theories on the attention of women and their focus on many outside factors during sex, Tantric Theory states that even if she wanted to, she would not have the ability to turn her focus inward. The belief is that women are unable to get in touch with the sensations of their body or their sexual desires because they have been raised to always put those aside, thus never developing the skills to do so. If she is not able to get in touch with these parts of herself, she will have great difficulty reaching orgasm. This is because she will have difficulty actually feeling what she is feeling, what she likes and doesn't like, and what she wants her partner to do in order to give her an orgasm. She will likely even have difficulty reaching orgasm when she is alone for the same reasons.

The Tantric Theory also has a theory concerning men and their pleasure. It is believed that men generally have short and intense orgasms and that it is possible for them to have better and longer-lasting orgasms through the practice of mindfulness as well. Tantra focuses on teaching men to be able to prolong their orgasms and make them more all-encompassing as well as to extend their pleasure overall.

Tantric Sex has many techniques and methods for overcoming these challenges, and its main intention concerning women is to help them refocus their attention on themselves and their body's sensations. By refocusing on their bodies, it allows women to fully access the parts of their brain related to sexual arousal without just as equally activating the parts of their brain related to worry and concern for others.

The practice of Tantra, in general, involves being in touch with one's feelings and one's breath—almost like a meditation. Neotantra or Tantric Sex takes this idea and uses it in relation to sex. Sex with oneself or sex with a partner is done through a deep connection to oneself and one's partner. In order to do this, you practice being connected to yourself and your deeper feelings in order to feel all of the sensations in your body more easily and reach orgasm quicker and with more intensity.

Tantric Sex is so useful for couples, especially those who have been together for some time. At the beginning of your relationship, you were connected by lust, the exploration of each other, and excitement. Now, since you know each other so well, it can be hard to reach that same feeling of discovery in the bedroom. Tantric Sex can help you get there.

For men, Tantric Sex aims to help them to fully feel and enjoy their orgasms, to make them more intense and longer-lasting, and to make them build up much more before releasing. It teaches women to be more present in their pleasure and, as a result, their orgasms. Accomplishing these things as well as reaching a greater level of intimacy with your partner is sure to bring you to a new level of connection within your relationship, no matter how long you have been together. Devote yourselves to this practice over time (it won't happen overnight), and it will give you something to work towards as a couple and get you excited about sex with each other again.

Tantric Massage Techniques

Tantric massage is a very common way to practice Tantric Sex. This massage can be on one of the genital areas such as the testicles, the penis, the vulva, the nipples, and so on, or it can be done on the head or shoulders. The intention here, regardless of where the massage takes place, is to focus on your breathing and get into a state of mindfulness. When you can do this, you will feel each of your partner's fingers, putting gentle pressure into your skin and the sensations that this produces inside of you. By being in this state during the massage, it is a great way to get your body ready to experience sex in a deeper way, which will greatly increase the chances and intensity of orgasm.

Yoni Massage

A Yoni Massage is a vaginal massage that is intended to open up the woman to her sexuality, her pleasure, and her sexual desires. As a partner, you can perform this type of massage for your woman to unlock her repressed sexual energy and help her to get in touch with it.

This can be done in a variety of ways, but the position we are going to discuss is a Hot Water Yoni Massage. Begin by setting the ambiance, either in the bathroom with a bathtub or around your jacuzzi. Set up some candles, some flowers, or anything that will make the surroundings relaxing and calm. Begin by having her breathe deeply and focus on her body and its sensations. You can get into the water with her for added intimacy. Begin by slowly and gently massaging around her entire vulva and her clitoral area. The key to this type of massage is to do everything very slowly. Begin to massage her clitoris slowly and not with the intention of making her come. When ready, and with lots of waterproof lube, slide one finger inside of her vagina and gently begin massaging the upper wall. Here is where her G-spot is located. Encourage her to express and release any sounds she naturally makes. Move your finger in a circular motion slowly and with your other hand, massage her pelvic area and clitoris. This connects the inner with the outer. Continue to do this and let the experience unfold with no end goal in mind. If she reaches orgasm, she can do so, but if she doesn't, she can just enjoy the pleasures that she is getting from your massage. As discussed earlier, this massage is intended to reconnect a woman with her pleasure and allow her to focus on herself and her body. After this massage, she will feel more in touch with her body, and if penetrative sex ensues, both of you will feel even more pleasure and intensity of orgasms because of how engorged and activated her vagina and clitoris will be. After doing this practice for some time, either with you or on her own, she will be more in tune with her body all of the time and not just when doing this practice. This will lead to stronger orgasms overall and hotter sex for both of you.

Whatever direction this takes afterward (sex or no sex), being able to connect with your partner in this physical and energetic way will be beneficial to your sex life and your relationship as a whole. It can help the woman to reach orgasm during penetration because both of your bodies will have formed a deep connection where the pleasure is able to build both independently and together. Both of you will be in touch with your own and each other's bodies while also being comfortable, allowing your body to feel whatever it may feel, and being present enough in the moment to welcome this.

Tantra is an ancient practice that has been helping couples to reconnect for decades. While you may not see yourself as someone who practices specific meditation or spiritual techniques of any sort, or if you tend to relate to more modern ideas, you may be wondering if Tantra is for you. The way that Tantra has been incorporated into sex and sexuality is actually quite a modern approach to Tantra, but nevertheless, there is a reason that its beliefs and techniques remain virtually unchanged after all this time.

Chapter 2. Benefits of Tantric Sex

Tantric Sex will help in uniting two individuals and help in their otherworldly, passionate, and mental association. In this part, you will find out about the different advantages that Tantric Sex has on offer.

Individual Growth

Tantric Sex helps in expanding the closeness remainder in a relationship. It additionally helps in the development of people also. An individual would have the option to develop intellectually, truly, just as profoundly. Tantric Sex helps in arousing Kundalini in ladies, and this takes into account her ladylike nature to radiate through. She will begin to sparkle and have a more uplifting standpoint and demeanor towards life. The male vitality, Shiva, encourages a man to tackle all his manly vitality through harmony and internal quality.

Exploring the Limits

Quick ones and self-pleasuring strategies are turning out to be very basic nowadays, and individuals are usually passing up the advantages that important and cherishing sex can give. This blocks a person from investigating their sexual cutoff points. Tantric Sex can help turn this around. Tantric Sex would help a person in understanding their actual sexuality and their sexual cutoff points. At the point when a couple participates in Tantric Sex, they structure a profound and significant bond that permits each partner to encounter sexual ecstasy. Tantric Sex can be thought of as a collaboration where each partner helps the other reach and reel in incredible physical, enthusiastic, and sexual delight that can be experienced by both.

Heightened Orgasms

The climaxes accomplished through Tantric Sex are more remarkable than the normal ones. The different Tantric Sex positions referenced in this book will help you in accomplishing pivotal climaxes. The positions are planned with the end goal that they hit all the sweet spots and cause your body to sing. It is an overall thought that ladies can have a more elevated level of climax when contrasted with men; however, with Tantric Sex, the two people can accomplish a higher condition of climax.

Knowing What Works

When you have figured out how to get its hang, Tantric Sex can be pleasant and energizing. With each progressive meeting, you will improve comprehension of your sexuality, your triggers, and those of your partner. You will have the option to comprehend what you and your partner appreciate. When you have figured out how to recognize these delight focuses, you can begin invigorating them for accomplishing unadulterated sexual euphoria. The physical and mental bond that you would have built up with your partner would essentially rely upon them and reinforce over a period, and you will arrive at a phase where you, as a team, gotten subject to one another's sexual vitality for their pleasure.

Timed Bliss

You can time your climaxes with Tantric Sex. When an individual has figured out how to deal with their psyche just as their body, they can naturally fall into a synchronized example for accomplishing a shared climax. Another type of vitality is produced, and it moves through every one of them when they have coordinated climaxes. This intensifies the connection between couples. Lessons of Tantric Sex propose that remaining associated after a sexual demonstration will help in fortifying the bond that is framed.

Monogamy

It is a prevalent view that Tantric Sex can help a couple in remaining together for the remainder of their life expectancy. At the point when two people have figured out how to produce a bond that encourages them to interface on a more profound plane, they become subordinate. This reliance can't be impersonated or reproduced with any other person. At the point when the recurrence of the meeting begins to expand, at that point, the connection between the people likewise begins to extend and fortify.

Health Benefits

Tantric Sex helps in advancing great wellbeing. Ladies will profit by this since it will help in making their period more ordinary, and this, thus, encourages them to keep their bodies fit as a fiddle. Tantric Sex helps in delivering certain male hormones that produce more advantageous and more grounded sperms, consequently expanding the couple's fruitfulness. A full-body climax helps in powering the body cells and helps in expanding their solidarity to battle ailment along these lines expanding the resistance. Ladies and men who have Tantric Sex will, in general, look more youthful because this is an extraordinary pressure buster. It likewise adds another sparkle to the face. Aside from all the different advantages that it has to bring to the table for everybody, Tantric Sex can additionally help in delivering serotonin that helps with keeping discouragement under control. A climax helps in delivering serotonin that helps in keeping cortisol under control and improves a person's mind-set.

Inhibitions

It additionally helps in causing an individual to get familiar with their body and be more alright with their body and that of their partner. The vast majority nowadays will, in general, get incredibly cognizant about their bodies, and these feelings of dread that they harbor prevent them from altogether appreciating sex, and they wind up having unremarkable sex. When you let go of the dread of being judged and have acknowledged your body for how it is, at that point, you will have the option to genuinely give up and relish the experience, as it was intended to be appreciated. If you let go of every one of these apprehensions, you can appreciate physical delight. Relinquishing your restraints will make sex more pleasant. Tantric Sex energizes this deserting.

Power Struggle

On the off chance that you follow the mainstream TV arrangement *Game of Thrones*, at that point, you will recollect the scene where Daenerys Targaryen breaks all the standards and chooses to assume responsibility for pleasuring her alpha-male spouse, Khal Drogo. Drogo objects from the start, yet then he gives in once he understands how pleasurable it truly is. About sex, usually, individuals will, in general, face an inward force battle. People both will, in general, like the sentiment of being in charge, though indicating that they are in charge can harm a relationship. There is a contrast between being in charge and appreciating shared Tantric Sex. Tantric Sex will help in taking out this difficult inside and out. Tantric Sex gives the equivalent capacity to both the partners, and the various positions will help in permitting both the gatherings to be in control, and they can give every delight to the other individual with no limitations.

Happiness

Tantric Sex helps in diverting all the positive types of vitality, and this will help in making the individual very upbeat. Since it is profoundly, genuinely, and truly fulfilling, an individual would be upbeat in every one of these viewpoints. The profound association that it lets you structure with holiness makes a difference.

Increased Love

There are a huge number of musings that experience your psyche at some random purpose of time. We will, in general, consider various individuals, not really our partners. It's very basic these days for couples to sever their connections on the affection that they aren't feeling "the adoration" any longer. Tantric Sex won't just assistance you in cherishing yourself, yet it will likewise help you in adoring your partner. It helps in building up a sustaining relationship that helps in shared development. This sort of solidarity of feeling makes the relationship stronger.

Empowers Both Men and Women

Most ladies will, in general, experience the ill effects of low confidence. They have become tormented with musings and sentiments that their bodies are flawed. They might not have the ability to disapprove of their partner while occupied with a sexual demonstration. They may not be really ready to have intercourse yet are constrained into it due to their powerlessness to state no. They probably won't express their actual emotions and wants uninhibitedly, and this decreases the joy that they experience. As per the lessons of Tantric Sex, ladies are dealt with like goddesses, and they are showered with the consideration and the regard that they merit. Moreover, even men are tormented with various issues concerning how they see themselves. Most men stress over how they are performing, regardless of whether they can fulfill their partner if their endurance is sufficient, et cetera. Rather than getting a charge out of the demonstration, they are frequently stressed over how long they can last.

At the point when they follow the lessons of Tantric Sex, they will feel enabled since their bodies are respected as the vessels of God. This will make them more certain and open to new encounters without living with those apprehensions and hindrances.

Immense Satisfaction

There are times when you may have engaged in sexual relations and felt that something was absent in it. You may feel that there's no energy or sentiment. This will, in general, occur since sex doesn't go past intercourse. It stops at the physical demonstration. Sex alone doesn't do anything for a relationship. Tantric Sex is more pleasurable since it helps in framing a passionate connection between partners rather than a straightforward physical bond. At the point when an individual has sincerely put resources into a demonstration, it turns out to be more pleasurable and charming. At the point when both are, it gets mysterious.

Alleviates Depression

Consider Tantric Sex as your guide. It will help you in defeating wretchedness and even nervousness. Individuals are typically too tired to even think about eating or rest nowadays. This unleashes destruction on their day by day plan. Tantric Sex will help you in handling the issues referenced previously. After a meeting of Tantric Sex, you will feel revived and reenergized, and this freshly discovered harmony and vitality will loosen up your body and quiet your psyche, consequently disposing of all the pointless strains that continue focusing on you. Tantric Sex is far beyond simply sex!

Chapter 3. The Basics of Tantric Sex

When you begin to follow the path of Tantric Sex, you begin to find a change in yourself. You find yourself changing how you view yourself and how you view the world. You find yourself looking at relationships that will last a lifetime. Through your journey, you will learn that every man and woman has a certain level of divinity in them. You will start to view sex as a sacred act instead of just a physical act. You will also learn to love deeper and find that you are soaring to different levels of bliss.

You will only have a successful journey when you relieve yourself from any preconceived notions. You should not think of what you need to do and what your lover must do to please you. When you read this, you will be able to identify new ideas about yourself and also embrace new ideas about yourself. You will also learn how to have great sex!

You will learn the basic concepts of Tantric Sex and identify new exciting ways to live and love.

The Yin and the Yang: Which Is Male, and Which Is Female?

You must be familiar with the stereotypes that men are from Mars and women are from Venus. This implies that men are assertive and extremely powerful, while women are soft and fragile, who are only fit for nurturing. There are other stereotypes that men do not show any feelings whatsoever, while women have a plethora of emotion that is ready to unleash itself in a second. It has also been said that women do not take credit for the work that they do since being outgoing is something only men are familiar with. Over the last few years, there has been a drastic change in the way men and women think.

Tantric Sex is a firm follower of the fact that men and women do have opposite characteristics. This is the elementary principle of the Tantra. The eastern theories claim that Yin represents feminism, while Yang represents masculinity. But there is no concrete proof that a woman cannot have Yang characteristics or that a man cannot have Yin characteristics. Rather than viewing men and woman as two entities, you should begin to focus on the energies. The Tantra believes in the amalgamation of these two energies.

Shiva and Shakti

The most common image of the Yin and the Yang is the Hindu divine couple Lord Shiva and Goddess Shakti. Lord Shiva represents the entire universe since he is considered the creator, and Goddess Shakti represents the root of all energy. The union of the two deities creates a longing in you and every other human being to be treated like a god or a goddess. You will learn to worship your partner as a god or a goddess.

The male energy that is found in Lord Shiva represents ecstasy, while the energy in Goddess Shakti represents wisdom. This magical combination is what helps a person attain enlightenment. This perfect couple is always represented in numerous entwined positions—either dancing or embracing or standing together. There are other positions where Goddess Shakti is wrapped around Lord Shiva, with her legs propped around his hips. The dancing position by far is the most sacred since they are able to free their spirit, giving them a chance to attain enlightenment.

Understanding the Opposites

You may have made divisions amongst you and your partner. You have to first identify and understand these divisions to strike a balance between the opposite energies. There are quite a few stereotypical characteristics that you may relate to. You will have to identify those characteristics and make a note of them. You have to go from one extreme. You should ask your partner to do this too. You will then have to see how you can embrace the extreme characteristics that you and your partner have. You have to identify how you can strike a balance between the polarities that exist between you and your partner. You will have to identify the Yin to your partner's Yang and vice versa.

You might now wonder if it is true that opposites attract. Sit back and think for yourself. You will be able to answer this question on your own. Try analyzing your past relationships. See how you and your partner were different from each other. Identify whether the differences were complemented by each other. This will help you analyze your future relationships as well.

My Partner Is My Beloved

Tantra is not mad love but sacred love. You are honoring your partner and cherishing your partner while making love. You will shower unconditional love with your partner. When you are talking to your partner, use loving words like "darling" or "beloved." You will find that those little words have aroused feelings of love within your partner. Call your partner with the aforementioned loving words when talking about them in public. You might find it terribly strange to do so, but you will be sending out a message of love to the person you are speaking to.

The Desire Spectrum

You will find yourself with new views of desire. You may feel a desire every time you think of someone. You may comment on how you want a guy or how hot a girl is when you see them passing. You only feel these desires when you feel incomplete. Since you feel incomplete, you always want another person. You find yourself feeling needy and feeling wanted. But when you do get the person you want, you begin to want something more. You want someone prettier, more interesting, and sometimes someone richer. Through Tantric Sex, you will be able to detach yourself from superficial needs. This will help you create a healthier relationship with your partner.

You Feel Empowered to Say What You Want!

When you find yourself empowered, you are able to set boundaries both during sex and in life in general. You find yourself with a new level of self-esteem. In Tantric Sex, you OWN your body and your soul. When your partner wants you to enter you, he must ask for your permission. You should not be afraid and have to say yes or no as the situation demands. You have to stop and say that you do not want to be touched in a way that is not comfortable. You empower your partner when you speak the truth this way. You will be giving your partner the methods to use to please you. You have to be okay with how you are touched and how you feel.

Chapter 4. How Tantric Massage Should Be Performed

Tantric massage is consequently, in fact, a Tantric practice. It occurs naked, both for the ones who receive for the ones who give; nudity brings to a deeper feeling in getting the massage, joint with a sense of greater freedom. At the time of the treatment, the body's energies are stimulated to move better, also augmenting enjoyment. All this helps to develop the awareness of one's senses, to get to know each other better both from inside oneself and relative to the external world.

It thus becomes a great opportunity for meditation and expansion of the Self, continuous listening. From a technical point of view, Tantric Massage is expressed through an intense succession of manual skills designed to stimulate a meditative state through a more intense perception of physicality and sensory abilities without also avoiding genital stimulation. In this case, the genital stimulation is not aimed at providing a mere pleasure, but at treating the genitals as if they were (and are) any other part of the body, without usually avoiding them morally, leaving this body part so important. It is the center of primary sexual energy, not integrated with the rest of the body, also because the Tantra Massage focuses on widespread body pleasure and not just genital pleasure. However, Tantric Massage is not a method of implying an erotic relationship that is not so.

The human body is a totality, and everything is sacred, worthy of attention. There are no areas closed by the Spirit. Unfortunately, in our society, bad information and education are still widespread.

The deep meaning of massage is, therefore, global body integration, which allows us to finally feel united and recomposed in the heart as well as in the perceived corporeality.

The Tantric Massage cannot be carried out in series; it will change and transform from person to person since everyone has a different body and energy. In addition, even performed on the same person, the massage will never be the same because the energy will change with it from time to time.

What Type of Sensations Can the Tantric Massage Bring?

Sensations and effects are entirely subjective; since it is a liberation of one's energy and a deep recognition of oneself and one's individuality, it is clear that perceptions and effects are varied. In general, however, it can be said that a constant sense of liberation, peace, harmony, and rebalancing can be observed as constant effects.

Tactile stimulations, which affect the psychosomatic aspects of the massage, powerful alternating techniques, delicate touches, sacred rituals, sensual and meditative manual skills, activation of the chakras, and other subtle energies.

It should be noted that this is due to the fact that Tantric Massage is not a standard technique but an expression of attention conveyed by Tantrika. In fact, the massage technique often hides traps that cage the holistic operator in patterns, which are ill-suited with Tantric Massage.

The Tantra Massage can be carried out seriously only by those who are in the Via del Tantra: someone who has realized the essence of Tantra in their life, and since Tantra is experiential, it cannot be explained but only experienced and perceived personally. It cannot be studied; if anything, it can be a direct transmission; one could say a kind of "initiation" that can only happen with particular Masters.

The spiritual aspect in Tantric Massage can be expressed through intimate and silent listening, inner purity, the action that comes from the Heart, the awareness of the "Sacrality of the body" perceived as the temple of the Soul.

The Tantric touch is a tool that develops awareness that is the true and only goal of Tantra. The Tantra ritual massage is both experiential and meditative, designed to awaken the body's consciousness by helping to reconnect with our unconscious where the traces of our most deeply rooted conditionings reside.

Tips on How to Perform a Tantric Massage

A Tantric Massage can perform the following three phases:

In the first phase, we focus on meditation, creating in a suitable and intimate place, such as the bedroom, a welcoming environment, with soft lights, incense, practicing exercises of breathing, and reciting mantras.

The second stage concentrates on gentle and round massages that are done on the face and body, starting in the legs until the arms, going through the pubic area, the back, the neck, and the head, with sweet touches along the channels of life energy, the chakras, and nadis. A lukewarm and delicate carrier oil is used, such as coconut oil.

The Use of Oil

Using essential oils for the body will make Tantra Massage be even more effective and pleasant. This, in addition to an atmosphere full of incense and relaxing music. The oils good for Tantric Massage must be applied once you start to touch the recipient's body and can be made on lavender, mint, calendula, basil, cinnamon, rosemary, sage, sandalwood, pine. Those are all fragrances known to stimulate blood circulation and promote muscle relaxation. Both for Tantra Massage and for other types of oriental massages, essential oils are used since they have a strong penetration capacity in the body; in particular, coconut oil, which is aroma-free and does not irritate the skin.

Chapter 5. How to Make a Tantric Massage to a Woman—Yoni Massage

The Yoni massage has recently gained some fans. The word Yoni, for those who do not know, has a Sanskrit origin and means the same as the female genital organ.

Some refer to the woman's vagina as a "sacred temple." This is because the vagina is a very erogenous zone and deserves to be exploited in different ways, overcoming the spheres of oral sex and simple penetration. In the philosophy of Tantra, Yoni is considered with respect and love for followers.

The main goal of the Yoni massage is to make the woman deeply relax and experience sensations that she has never experienced in her entire life. In addition, the massage that is performed by men's fingers further extends the degree of intimacy between the couple, therefore essential for the health of the relationship. The partner of the massage is called "donor," to give the woman all the pleasure she deserves and should never expect anything in return.

Know that to do the Yoni massage in your partner; you have to be selfless; you should never do the massage—which can also generate multiple orgasms in the woman and expect something in return or a pleasure. Sex after a massage can also happen, but usually, this is not the rule, especially if the woman enjoys and is already exhausted with so much pleasure.

Although this is not a sexual technique for men, it can be very pleasant for him since he can see his partner up close as he has never seen before, trembling with so much heat and moaning like crazy. Which man has never thought of leaving a woman in this state, even with her powerful fingers? So, learn the Yoni massage technique and apply it to your loved one!

Prepare the Environment

Before you start, you must be careful to prepare the environment. In Tantra, the place where sexual activities are given is very important because it directly affects the whole process and the mental state of each. Putting a half-light on the environment, smelling incensed flowers, lighting candles, arranging curtains, scarves, and colored cushions can create a totally favorable atmosphere for what will come.

Remember to put a silent ambient sound to balance the space. Humans are sensitive to the senses; therefore, the activation of the sense of smell, hearing, sight, and even touch can allow the experience to be more intense for the woman and increase her interaction with herself. Even as a donor, you will feel more relaxed in developing the technique.

First, a Nice Shower

One of the recommendations of the Yoni massage is to take a relaxing shower before proceeding step by step. The woman can bathe alone by simply lathering herself or throwing water, or you can participate in the bathroom by starting the ritual of connection and intimacy between you.

Try to make this moment something special, without haste, and try to enjoy each other's presence. This bath will bring more vigor to both, as well as disinfect the entire region you will explore.

Balanced Breathing

For Yoni massage to work, it is important that your breathing is synchronized. Hence, man and woman should seek a balance of breathing, a calm, regular, and calm breath. Shortness of breath shows insecurity, anxiety, or even excitement in advance, and the Yoni massage indicates that hormones are controlled, and the woman is completely relaxed, available, and confident with everything she will feel soon. Inhale and exhale together until you are in perfect harmony; if necessary, you can also do a yoga session before finding the balance you need.

Disconnect From Everything

You and your partner should be fully involved with each other, and with space, they have prepared for the activity. Therefore, it is recommended to forget everything outside of that space, all worldly and material things. Turn off the smartphone, laptop, close the door, unplug the intercom, the phone, close the windows, curtains and then immerse yourself in the universe you created. Obviously, not only material matters are important, but you two should also make an effort not to disperse concentration with thoughts about problems and other concerns from outside.

Placement

Make sure to make the woman comfortable. You can let her observe the massage, the movements you perform, and even your image to make it even more stimulated. She may want to keep her eyes closed so that she can feel all the vibrations more fully; it will depend on the choice of each.

The legs should be separated, and the knees bent in the typical position of a woman when she is about to give birth. Her genital organ must be fully exposed to you as a donor, who can sit in front of her to be able to perform all movements with ease and free access.

Start With the Massage

Start by massaging her legs, thighs, breasts, abdomen, and other regions before reaching the vagina. Pour a small amount of lubricant, which can be purchased in specialty stores and sex shops. Then squeeze the outer lip between your thumb and forefinger and slide up and down with slow and precise movements. Then, do the same movement on the inner lip, always calmly, getting the woman used to the touch. It is recommended that the couple maintain eye contact during the massage to intensify the sensation and exchange between the two.

Since the preference for intensity, speed, and pressure varies from woman to woman, the woman should tell the donor what she prefers while experiencing the sensations.

This will make it easier for the donor to find the right spot for his pleasure. But it limits the conversation since prolonged speech can be a factor in dispersing the massage.

Focus on the Clitoris

The clitoris is a complex structure, similar to the glans penis in the male sex. So, it is extremely sensitive and erogenous; it can be up to four times more sensitive than the glans penis, in fact. This is because it has between 6 and 8 thousand nerve endings, which helps to be one of the largest female pleasure generators.

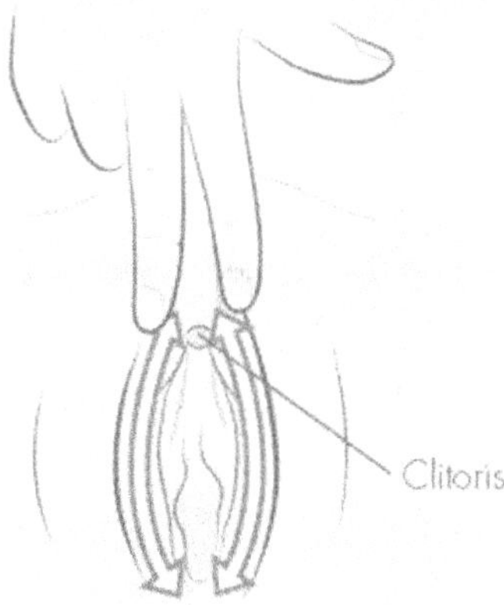

When massaging the clitoris, it is necessary to make circular movements clockwise and counterclockwise. Slowly insert the middle finger of your right hand into the vagina and make various movements—using your right hand has everything to do with the polarity of Tantra.

G-Spot or "Holy Place"

Massage the inside of the vagina with your finger, varying the speed, depth, and pressure. With your finger still inside the vagina, do the "come here" movement over and over again. In this area, you will be in contact with a spongy tissue that is located under the public bone and behind the clitoris.

Finalization

At the same time, you can use the little finger of the right hand to insert it into the woman's anus, obviously, if she accepts. So, you can extend her feeling of pleasure with the Yoni massage. In the meantime, you can use your free hand (left hand) to massage the breast, abdomen, or clitoris. The woman, completely sensitive to touch, can even cry due to the sensations, wince, and have multiple orgasms. Just stop when she asks.

How to Make a Tantric Massage to a Man?

Unlike a conventional erotic massage, the Tantric Massage of the penis and lingam does not only aim to achieve ejaculation to your partner but to stimulate the energy of this important erogenous zone to experience pleasure and to stimulate a sexual connection from a different perspective. Having made this philosophical-spiritual premise, let's go into more detail on how to do a Tantric Massage to a man.

1. To begin doing a Tantric Massage to a man, create an ideal environment for relaxation. Also, choose a moment of calm in which you know that you will hardly be interrupted because this

massage will not be a quick meeting, so it is good that both participants immerse themselves at the moment without looking at the clock—light up the house with aromatic candles and incense. Create an atmosphere that promotes calm and pleasure.

2. Play to stimulate and excite your partner as you usually do, but relying on all your senses: your eyesight, stripping you gradually and seductively; touch, letting it caress your body and caress it in turn; the taste, with the flavor of kisses; the sense of smell with the smell of your lover's skin and yours and finally with hearing, thanks to a whole series of words and expressions of the erotic vocabulary that you know.

3. Before starting a Tantric Massage for a man, it is important to know all the sensitive points of your partner's genitals, as well as the whole penis. Stimulate the pleasure potential that can be obtained by stimulating the testicles, massaging the scrotum, and stimulating the perineum, all extremely important areas for carrying out this massage.

4. Lubrication is essential for Tantric lingam or penis massage. Use gentle oil like almond oil, which is a good conditioner that will give more delicacy to your movements, making the experience a series of incredible sensations for him.

5. For this Tantric Massage, you will have to use both hands; the movements will be ascending as indicated in the image and also descending but in a more delicate way. One of your hands will

massage the testicles, the scrotum, and the perineum, while the other will focus on the penis from the base of the shaft to the glans, always keeping the rhythm and using your hands in their entirety. You have to take the penis and testicles with the whole palm, gently so as not to hurt, but confidently at the same time in order to generate pleasure.

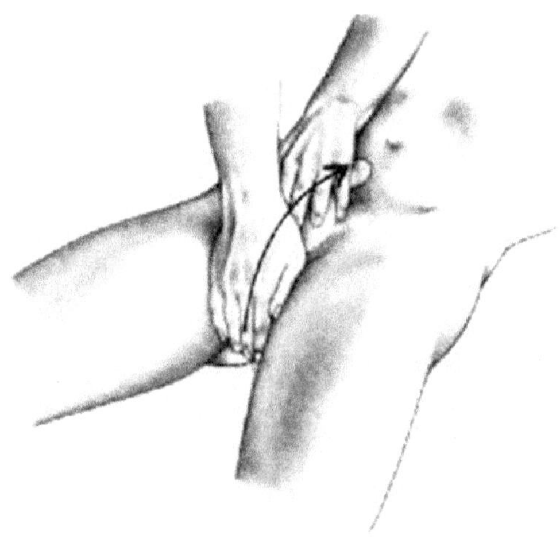

To do a Tantric Massage to a man, it is important that you yourself let yourself go with pleasure in doing the Tantric Massage and infuse energy that your boy will perceive immediately. Try to be creative, too; let the sexual energy permeate you to make your partner enjoy it too. Do not limit yourself, do not think if you are doing it well or badly; take advantage of this practice to increase intimacy and create new complicity.

Chapter 6. Tantric Sex and Men's Multiple Orgasms

One very important aspect of Tantric Sex is that it posits that climaxing during sex is not the same as ejaculating. If you are prone to feeling empty and unsatisfied even after you ejaculate, you might not be experiencing an orgasm. Hence, it is not necessary for a male to ejaculate in order to experience the sexual pleasures of orgasm.

By applying methods of orgasm control that are present within Tantric philosophy, you will be able to experience multiple orgasms and even orgasms that last incredibly long amounts of time.

A particular Tantric technique that you might be interested in would allow you to orgasm for several hours at a time. However, before you are able to achieve this level of Tantric sexual prowess, you are going to have to practice orgasm control within the confines of Tantric philosophy.

This is a form of skimming the waters without actually going inside for a swim. There are three strategies that can help you to do this:

Get Ready to Kegel

The pubic muscles, which are essentially the muscles in your groin, are the muscles that control your sex. They are basically included in the muscles you'd use to hold it in if you have to pee. Strengthening these pubic muscles to a certain degree can allow you to control your orgasm, and the most efficient method of strengthening these muscles is to do Kegels.

Kegels are very basic exercises that do not require you to put in an extraordinary effort. Simply clench your pubic muscles around two dozen times before or after each meal. However, remember not to go overboard with this exercise.

After a few weeks of regularly performing this exercise, try to prolong the length of time during which you hold the squeeze. Initially, go for two to three seconds per squeeze, but your ultimate goal should be about ten seconds per squeeze. This exercise will help you prolong your orgasm and will also keep you from climaxing too soon.

Keep Your Cool

This may sound odd to you, but the best thing you can do to prolong your sex is to stay calm if an orgasm starts coming on before you want it to just slow down your breathing and stop thrusting.

Keep in mind that this might cause some awkwardness between you and your partner, so make sure that you keep communicating. Don't be shy; just let her know that you are trying not to come, and she will understand. After all, the longer you last before you have an orgasm, the longer she has to build up to your orgasm!

Take It Slow

When you begin to have sex with your lover, remember to take it slow at first. The slower the sex is, the sweeter the orgasm because the buildup will be a lot more intense.

Regulate your breathing, and when you feel the orgasm coming on, try to calm yourself down by taking a deep breath and then clench your pubic muscles.

Once the orgasm recedes somewhat, it is safe to begin thrusting again. Repeat this process as much as possible, stopping and clenching at regular intervals. This will allow you to build excitement within your partner to incredible levels!

Eventually, you are going to want your climax; otherwise, the sex would end up becoming frustrating. This is when your orgasm control will come into play.

Once you are close to orgasm, and this time, you actually want to climax, let it happen and then clench your pubic muscles while it is happening. This will prevent you from ejaculating but would give you the full pleasure of the orgasm that you are experiencing.

If you fail at this technique initially, don't take it too hard. It is actually a fairly difficult technique to master, but with a bit of practice, you will be stopping your orgasms in no time, allowing you to have hours of sex!

The Female Orgasm

Don't worry. Tantra is just as aware of the problems women face during sex as it is of males. This is why there are sexual practices in this spiritual way of life for women too!

A common saying in Tantric philosophy is that the most powerful organ of sex that a woman possesses is her mind. This is because her arousal can often be dampened by negative emotions that would get in the way of her lust. These thoughts, emotions like anxiety or anger, or guilt, can have a profound impact on your sex because they would distract your partner from the act of lovemaking.

Hence, it is important to place less of an emphasis on the theatrics of lovemaking and more on what your woman is feeling. However, this important piece of information is not enough to allow you to give your woman the mind-blowing orgasms that she deserves, so listed below are some techniques that you can apply.

Clitoral Stimulation

What most men are practically clueless about is the fact that women are not all that turned on by penetration. The act is erotic in and of itself, and it provides some sexual stimulation, but the clitoris provides the majority of sexual stimulation.

Hence, it is very important that you stimulate the clitoris if you want your woman to achieve orgasm. Be gentle in the way that you stimulate the clitoris, and be patient. Overdoing it can cause women discomfort.

Additionally, don't pressure your partner to orgasm, as this would stress her out and completely turn her off from the sex.

The G-Spot

In Tantra, there is what is called a sacred spot within a woman's vagina. This spot is a couple of inches within the vaginal canal on the top. This sacred spot is often called the g spot and is the key to giving your partner extremely explosive orgasms.

Place a finger into your partner's vagina and attempt to feel for the spot at the top of the vaginal canal. You will feel it as being about half the size of a penny with a crumpled surface that is almost like the ripples inside your own mouth.

The vast majority of women can have excellent orgasms induced by stimulating this spot, with many of these women even ejaculating, which is a very rare occurrence that happens only when an earth-shaking orgasm happens.

The g spot, or sacred spot, is a nexus of powerful Tantric energy. It is believed by some to be a source of kundalini energy. Stimulating this spot releases that energy in a way that no other pressure point in the body is able to release. This energy shoots up within your body, activating your kundalini and all of your other chakras for a fraction of a second.

Hence, a g spot orgasm is a source of not only pleasure but immense power as well!

Chapter 7. Teachings of Tantric Sex

Let us take a closer look at the teachings of Tantric Sex that will help in improving not only the level of intimacy but also the sexual pleasure that you and your partner experience. This will have a positive effect on your relationship. When these teachings are made use of in the proper manner, then it will put you a step closer to achieving enlightenment. Each one of these teachings can be made use of in a sexual and non-sexual way.

Breathe

Remember to keep breathing. You probably would have understood by now the importance of breathing when it comes to Tantric Sex. It is not just about Tantric Sex; any of the teachings that have originated in the East, regarding the attainment of enlightenment, tend to place a great deal of importance on breathing. It is crucial that you understand the reason why this is done and the manner in which it is related to Tantra, as well as the spiritual development of an individual.

The answer to this is quite simple, every living thing breathes. We breathe all the time, and if we do stop breathing for prolonged periods of time, it will ultimately result in death or even unconsciousness. In this manner, it could be simply understood that breathing can be related to our state of consciousness. Think of the breath as energy. Every breath that we take fills our body with oxygen and takes away carbon dioxide in this process. This oxygen that we inhale is then supplied to different cells in the body. Oxygen and breathing are fundamental to the functioning of our bodies.

Breathing isn't a voluntary or conscious function. It is something that our body has been designed to do. You might never pay any attention to the way you are breathing, but you never really stop breathing when you are alive. Isn't it intimidating how our life depends on a function that we don't even do voluntarily?

It is quite interesting to note the benefits of conscious and regulated breathing can have on different aspects of your life, including your sex life. It is common that while people are engaged in any sexual activity, they tend to hold their breath; this isn't a known function. Every time you get excited, you might notice that you tend to hold your breath. You probably hold onto your breath without even realizing that you are doing so. When you stop breathing, this will disrupt the flow of energy in your body as well. Making breathing a conscious act while engaged in sex will help you in learning to control your energy and the movement of energy in your body. This teaching of Tantra is all about taking breaths in a relaxed and calm manner. Let your breath flow slowly through your body. If you want to achieve a full-body orgasm, then you will have to make sure that your breathing is deep and even. When you start focusing on this, you will realize that you can climax more easily.

Relax

The tension in your muscles and body will act as an obstruction in a manner that is similar to shallow breathing. The muscular tension that you tend to experience when you are engaged in any sexual activity is not a conscious one. One of the principles of Tantric Sex is that you will need to be aware of this muscular tension that exists in your body and so that you are aware of all the different muscles that are being held up due to tension. You do require a little bit of tension for facilitating movement in the body and also for holding up the body, but that's it. Muscular tension isn't required in every part of the body.

If you start making the decision of tensing up your muscles a conscious one, then you will notice that you are probably tensing up a few muscles in your body unnecessarily while having sex. For instance, a man might end up tensing all his muscles while receiving oral sex. Whereas he's simply supposed to let go and enjoy the attention being showered by his partner, instead, he is tensing up the muscles in his torso and legs. In such a case, all the extra tension is unnecessary, and this simply obstructs the free flow of energy in the body. Focus your attention on relaxing all these tensed muscles. Focus on your breathing and enjoy the sexual warmth that is flowing through your body.

It Sounds That Can Help

Sounds are crucial when it comes to the movement of energy in the body. Some people may not be comfortable, or they might even be conscious of the sounds that they make when aroused. These considerations shouldn't be taken seriously while engaging in Tantric Sex. Let go of all the inhibitions that are holding you back. Express yourself as freely as you want to. There is no restriction apart from the ones that you have imposed on yourself. Make all the sounds that you feel like making. These sounds are involuntary reactions to the pleasure that you are experiencing, and they are connected with the emotions and sensations that you are experiencing. If you are silent or quiet, then the movement of sexual energy in your body gets slow. When you are vocal in expressing what you are feeling, the energy starts to move in the body. Tantric Sex is all about awakening the dormant sexual energy that is present within the body and then making use of it for achieving enlightenment. Well, how will the energy move when you are anxious about something as trivial as the way you sound?

Eye Contact Is Essential

This might sound like an obvious thing. Well, it does enhance the overall sexual experience. Looking at your partner while engaged in any sexual act will make the experience more intense eye contact doesn't mean that you stare wistfully into your partner's eyes. Move over to the longing look love-struck puppy has in its eyes. We are talking about some serious X-rated gazing, so get ready for it. This will help you attain some extra intimacy. For getting started, you and your partner can find a comfortable spot to sit so that you both will be able to look into each other's eyes. Take a moment to gather your thoughts; usually, a deep breath will do the trick for you. Once you feel that you are ready, you can open your eyes and gaze into your partner's eyes. Allow your partner the access to see you, your true self, sans any pretenses, and in a similar manner, you can gaze at them. This might feel a little stupid initially, but it will prove to be quite effective.

Allow yourself to communicate through your eyes and not just your genitals. You can let your eyes wander over each other's bodies. Let your partner see the lust in your eyes and the wanton abandonment. Nothing would be a better turn on than knowing that your partner desires you and needs you. In the manner that sounds and touch can communicate, in the same way, you can communicate a lot more by making use of just your eyes alone. This will help you both communicate with each other in an earnest manner.

Pay Attention

Energy flows in the body according to your attention. You will need to concentrate on this flow of energy in your body. If you want to experience a full-body orgasm, then the energy in your body should spread to every single cell. You will have to start paying some extra attention to the highly sexualized feelings that you want to experience throughout your body. If a woman wants to enjoy a vaginal orgasm, then she will need to focus on prying out the dormant sexual energy that is present within her and coax it to move freely in her body. You can make use of the other principles of Tantra for focusing your attention. For drawing out the energy and directing it towards the spot that you want it to go to, then you will need to visualize the same. Picture this energy moving from its resting place to the place where you want to experience a pleasure. The principles of Tantra suggest that energy needn't be confined to only one part of the body, and that is, in fact, should be moving throughout the body.

Always Be Present

The basic principle of all teachings is the need to be present at the moment. The present doesn't imply being present physically. It means being present mentally as well. You will have to be present at the moment. Don't let your mind or thoughts wander anywhere, and don't fantasize about anything else apart from the activity that you are involved in at the moment. Be present at the moment with your partner, and be aware of what is happening.

Exploration of Your Senses

Tantra is an ancient art, and it's been around for centuries. It is crucial to take note of the fact that Tantra isn't just about improving the physical quality of having intercourse, but it is also about enhancing the emotional experience. All your sensory organs tend to take part in your sexual experience. Sex isn't an isolated process. Therefore, Tantra is all about improving your sensory experience, as well. If one of your senses has been compromised then, the other senses tend to become sensitive.

Aim for a Full Body Orgasm

Who wouldn't want to have an orgasm? A full body orgasm does sound tempting, doesn't it? So, without wasting any time, let us get started with this fascinating concept.

One manner in which you can condition your body to have a full body orgasm is by practicing the build-up to an impending orgasm and then letting it subside without giving in to the pleasure. You will have to drive your partner to the brink of an orgasm and then let it fade away without letting them climax. Once you let it subside, you will have to start building it up again and let it fade away again. Use all your willpower and keep playing at it for as long as you possibly can.

The Journey Counts

Orgasms are wonderful, but Tantric Sex isn't about simply achieving an orgasm. It is about delaying your orgasm for a while longer to receive better results. An orgasm can be thought of as a wonderful by-product of engaging in Tantric Sex. Tantric Sex is more spiritual and sacred than regular sex. It is the union of the opposing sexual energies present in the partners. The pressure of having to achieve an orgasm tends to take away the pleasure of participating in a sexual act. This stress is quite harmful, and it has a negative impact on a person's performance. The journey in Tantric Sex is almost as important as a result. Orgasm isn't the main aim. It is about enjoying your body and your partner as well.

Chapter 8. Tantric Sex Is Better Than the Sex You're Having

Reasons Why Tantric Sex Is the Better Sex

There is more to Tantra than meets the eye. Tantric Sex is just but a single aspect of Tantra, and if you're wondering why you should begin adopting this approach to sex, you'll be pleased to discover there are many reasons why. Whether you're looking to make a better connection, improve your sex life, or just trying to shake up your relationship, once you set foot down this powerful sacred sexual pathway, you won't want to go back to the way it used to be.

Once you've decided to embrace Tantric Sex in your life, the old routines and habits need to be tossed out the window. You're beginning anew with a fresh mindset, with a focus on not just enjoying sex but also enjoying the freedom of being able to express your pleasure. Powerful orgasms (although that isn't the main goal, mind you), orgasms that last longer, multiple orgasms, enhanced intimacy levels, and better sex life overall are some of the many wonderful benefits that await you.

- **It makes you feel more spiritual**—Spirituality is not about being religious; it is about getting in touch with your soul and what truly matters in your life. Tantra opens you to a higher connection between you and your spiritual side. Being spiritual shifts your perspective to focus on the things that should matter most to you, leads you away from being too focused or consumed about the materialistic aspects of this world we are so often caught up with.

- **It gets rid of the pressure to "perform"**—Porn has led to a lot of misconceptions about what sex should be. Porn is not bad per se, but it can make you feel pressured to live up to those unrealistic expectations that you see on screen. We fail to remember that at the end of the day, what you see on screen is nothing more than performance. Purely for entertainment purposes. Tantra helps you eliminate some of that pressure by acting as the "anti-porn." Instead of focusing on living up to expectations, Tantra slows things down with movements that teach you to appreciate being in the moment with your partner. This is someone you love, and you should take the time to show them that love. Think about this moment when it is just the two of you and no one else. Gaze lovingly into their eyes and think about all the reasons why you love them for who they are.

- **It teaches you to accept yourself for who you are**—The person you are right at this moment is the person you are bringing to the Tantric experience you have with your partner. Embracing yourself for who you are. We may not admit it out loud; many of us are afraid of letting someone else see our true selves in case they don't like what they see. Tantra teaches you to look deep into your soul and into your heart, and because Tantra is about focusing on your energy, it makes it impossible for you to hide from the truth any longer.

- **It encourages communication**—Do you listen to your partner during sex? Do they listen to you? You both will once you begin the art of Tantric Sex since mindfulness is a big part of making this work. It encourages you to communicate when you slow it down and talk to each other and focus on what feels good as you touch each other. Couples are encouraged to be honest and as specific as possible. As your partner touches you, think about what that sensation feels like. Does it feel good? Let them know. Would you prefer something else? Let them know. Tantric Sex is about getting out of your head and turning your attention towards your body instead.

- **It teaches you to explore your limits**—Self-pleasuring techniques and quickies have taken away the meaning of what a sexual experience filled with love can do for you. When you miss out on that, it hinders you from exploring your sexual limits. Tantric Sex, of course, aims to turn that around by helping you understand your true sexuality. Couples who engage in Tantric Sex form a deep, meaningful bond, and it is this bond that allows both parties to experience sexual bliss. You work together as a team to see how far you can push your limits, how much more pleasure you can attain, and the earth-shattering orgasms that follow will make your body sing like never before.

- **It promotes monogamy**—A deep bond that is formed with another is a bond that is not severed quite so easily. The kind of bond that you form with your partner during Tantric Sex is going to transcend the connection you had previously before you began this journey. The closer you grow, the deeper your feelings become, and when you feel such love and affection for another, the desire to look elsewhere for pleasure gradually fades away.

Tantric Sex is something that both men and women can benefit from. The rejuvenating effects that it has claims to bring with it several health benefits because of the way that it changes the body's chemistry. Aside from the benefits that were talked about above, Tantric Sex is even better than the sex you're having right now because of the individual benefits it has for men and women. There are unique ways in which men and women benefit from the art of Tantric Sex.

For women, Tantric Sex is going to nourish the body, infuse the woman with energy and touch her heart and soul completely. For women, these are the reasons why Tantric Sex is better sex:

- **The health benefits**—It empowers a woman's endocrine glands, stimulating it to produce more of the HGH hormone, more serotonin, testosterone, and even the DHEA hormone. The energy that flows throughout the woman's body during sex can help to detoxify her through each breath that she takes, even improving her cardiovascular and immune system. Breathing techniques and learning how to regulate breath alone, for example, is a way of improving your health by allowing more air into the body, which then helps to nourish all the muscles and tissue within the body.

- **Unlocks the elusive G-spot**—In Tantra, it is referred to as the sacred spot, the woman's most mysterious erogenous zone, which also happens to be the most potent. The G-spot is located approximately two to three inches up along the front wall of her vagina. In Tantric philosophy, a lover who practices these ancient secret techniques can discover the body's direct sexual energy through its chakras.

- **It promotes feelings of empowerment**—Images of perfection perpetuated by the media have made it easy for women to forget that they are beautiful just the way that they are. Tantric Sex seeks to change that by helping women feel empowered by using their bodies to celebrate their desires. Women in Tantric Sex are treated with and given the respect and honor that they deserve. Their partners treat them with love and desire, worshipping their bodies like a goddess. This is beneficial for a woman's confidence and self-esteem.

- **It promotes healing**—Women, in general, is a lot more emotional than men. They wear their hearts on their sleeves, and past hurts, painful wounds, or traumatic experiences have a way of leaving behind a scar that never really fades away. Tantra opens the door for a woman to heal from within, rooted in the teachings that call for a woman to be loved, honored, and respected not just in sex but in life too.

As for men, Tantric Sex is the better sex for the following reasons:

- **It encourages men to understand their bodies better—** Through Tantra, men develop a greater understanding of their sexual energy and their bodies' response to pleasure. A lot of men do not pay enough attention to their bodies and their bodies' needs. With the focus so heavily concentrated on ejaculation, not enough attention is given to what makes them feel good. Tantra's practices will change all of that through mindfulness. This, in turn, encourages better communicative skills while in bed with their partner and can help derive more pleasure when they can translate what they need.

- **Sex becomes more than just what porn promotes—**Tantric Sex teaches both men and women that the act of sex is more than just two people having intercourse. That sex is something to be treated as a sacred act, something which has deep meaning and lasting effects, even long after the sex part is over. From a very early age, men and boys are conditioned away from prolonged pleasure. They are also led to believe that their sexuality is to be reserved and, at times, emotionless. This is exasperated by pornography that puts a false emphasis on ejaculation as the highest peak of pleasure and the primary goal. It is through Tantric Sex that men are awakened to the realization that sex should be treated with respect, cherished, and loved. It is one of the many reasons why it is so effective at deepening the bond between two people.

- **Achieving multiple orgasms**—It's no secret that most (if not all men) long to last longer and achieve multiple orgasms. A man can have whole-body, multiple orgasms, and can last for several minutes when Tantric Sex is involved. Part of Tantra's teachings involve semen retention practices and learning how to transfer that ejaculation intensity into orgasmic energy; a man can have just as many orgasms as a woman. Semen is the life-force of a man; it must be kept in the body for a man to maintain his health. The act of ejaculation greatly reduces the life-force running through a male organism and is immediately followed by a drop in energy, creating a depressive nature. When semen is retained in the body, it directly supports the brain and central nervous system. It improves function, reinstating energy and confidence, and eventually leads to multiple orgasms for the men too.

- **Minimizes the risk of depression**—Men and women are both susceptible to depression. Especially with the pressures, we face today. Tantra is one approach to minimizing the risk of depression because it encourages the elimination of negative energy and infuses both the mind and body with positive ones. The flow of energy movement and a heightened state of pleasure and bliss expels negative energy from the body.

Chapter 9. Improve Tantric Sex With These Tips

The principal motivation behind Tantra is to assist you with accomplishing splendid climaxes that you have been precluded in light of the fact that from securing your standard sexual practices. Notwithstanding, this doesn't imply that Tantra ought to be dealt with daintily. Consider Tantra an erotic exercise. Tantric Sex is viewed as more charming than going through hours together at the rec center, yet the measure of physical effort that your body encounters can be contrasted with that you may understanding while at the same time playing out any overwhelming activities.

Additionally, there are various degrees of Tantric Sex. Essentially, bouncing into Tantra with no experience or primer practice may improve your sexual coexistence, yet it is so much better when you participate in some type of pre-sex warm-up practice that will help in setting the mindset and working up some expectation concerning what is yet to come. There are a few manners by which you can heat up; however, perhaps the most ideal way that could be available is to give your partner a back rub and have your partner give you one also. This will extricate up your muscles, which is significant in light of the fact that solid muscles can hinder a full-body climax.

The back rub that you are providing for setting up your darling for Tantric Sex has some particular standards that are joined to it, alongside a system that is intended to uplift the sexual affectability and make the body progressively open to assist sexual incitement. Additionally, this back rub can be combined with a procedure that can be used on a lady to cause her to accomplish a climax. This will contribute extraordinarily to the nature of Tantric Sex in light of the fact that accepting one climax makes an individual patient for the following one, and this furnishes you with the fundamental open the door to coax your partner and draw out the sex.

The Use of Oil

The main thing that you need before you can give your sweetheart a pre-sex knead is oil. Oil is an incredible instrument that can be used if you need your back rub to be increasingly compelling. It helps in extricating the skin up and giving grease to your hands. If your hands can slide and coast easily over your darling's body all the more adequately, then it will likewise help in making the back rub increasingly sexy and causes in paving the way to real sex!

The best oil that you can use in a pre-sex rub is grape seed oil. This is because grape seed oil has a minimal number of individuals that are oversensitive to it and can be incredible for your skin. In this manner, by giving your sweetheart a grape seed oil rub, you will be helping him, or she gets milder skin too, and isn't this a fantastic special reward? You can generally include a couple of drops of your preferred scented or basic oil to make the experience far and away superior. Distinctive fundamental oils can be used, relying on the specific explanation behind which it is being used. For example, lavender can be used for unwinding and alleviating muscles; rose can be used for giving an increasingly erotic feel to the back rub.

If grape seed oil isn't accessible, go for whatever other oil that has been made with the end goal of back rubs.

The Technique

The primary thing that you should do is clearly begin spreading the oil over your sweetheart's body. Ensure that the oil is conveyed uniformly everywhere throughout the body, and remember that too little oil won't give sufficient oil and result in teasing. In any case, using an excess of would simply wind up getting chaotic, and this can be irritating. Attempt to locate the fair compromise! While you are spreading the oil over your partner's body, you will find that the skin ingests the oil rapidly. Thus, you should keep habitually spreading more oil over their body if the grease quits being adequate.

When the oil has been spread over your partner's body, the back rub can appropriately start. At first, it would be a smart thought, to begin with, essential pressure of the entirety of the significant muscles. The muscle you ought to go for while applying wide and vague pressure are the thigh muscles since this zone is normally under the most strain for the duration of the day.

When the muscles have been relaxed up in your partner's legs, you can move their back, the second-tensest region of the normal body. Simply apply pressure with your straightened palm, and make sure to speak with your partner as much as you can about what feels better and what is excruciating.

Attempt gently slapping territories that you feel are, as of now, free to invigorate blood courses in these zones. Recollect not to slap so hard that it harms except if your partner needs you to, obviously!

When you have finished this back rub and released up the significant muscle gatherings, the time has come to start centered pressure with the tips of your fingers and your clenched hands. There are explicit territories that you ought to focus on during centered pressure, and these zones are determined in the following segment.

Territories to Target

Bosoms: The bosoms are one specific territory of the human life systems that will, in general, draw in a great deal of consideration, and it so occurs that they are additionally an astounding wellspring of sexual incitement for some individuals. They likewise will, in general, have exceptionally thought purposes of strain that, when discharged, wind up, causing the individual to feel fantastically loose and quiet.

Along these lines, bosoms are clearly going to be one of the most significant zones of the body that you should target. Purposes of pressure here are most likely going to be on the lower half of the bosoms. It is significant that you search, attempting to discover the zone where the pressure exists.

This little wad of strain can be discovered right beneath the areola, and your partner may likely shout out when you hit this specific spot. In any case, don't confound this torment and stop the back rub. This torment is entirely charming, with numerous individuals contrasting it with the inclination one gets while scratching a tingle.

Something imperative to note while performing such a back rub is the source of these little wads of strain that are available in the body. They are not just strong pressure. Their root is more mystical than physical in nature.

You are, as of now, acquainted with the different chakras present in the body. In any case, you most likely don't know that these chakras are the significant stops in an immense system of energy that is streaming inside your body, vortices through which energy continually streams. However, there are certain circumstances where the progression of energy can get disturbed.

This typically occurs because of a less than stellar eating routine or a physical issue in a previous existence that may residually affect your body right now. Therefore, when you apply profound strain to these points, the energy begins to get discharged, consequently expelling the impediment that was formerly hindering the progression of energy in your body.

Discharging energy is agonizing and yet very charming in light of the fact that the progression of energy gives essentialness and expanded sexual affectability to your body. This implies when you knead these points, your partner is going to feel an extraordinary tingling vibe that will regress into a stimulating sensation as the blockage is expelled from the energy pathways in the body.

An ideal manner by which you can apply strain to this specific point is by pushing down using the tips of your fingers. Start by applying pressure and moving your hands in a round movement. This will discharge the energy blockage in a mellow and proficient manner. The round movement extricates up stuck energy and afterward permits your hand to move away to an alternate piece of the blockage, permitting the relaxed up energy to stream into the energy pathway without being impeded by the pressure of your fingers.

You can likewise apply serious strain to this point. This is exceptionally valuable since it will discharge energy from the blockage in a very serious way, and this will wind up opening your partner up for extraordinary sexual incitement.

Butt: This is another zone of the body that a great many people are stirred by. For reasons unknown, the butt is similarly as inclined to blockages in energy as bosoms seem to be, most likely in view of the extraordinary sum strain they experience when the individuals they are appended to spend by far most of their day sitting in an office. With the measure of sitting that we do, it is no big surprise that the pathways of energy in our derrieres wind up getting sponsored up.

The significant thing here is to feel your way around the territory. Blockages can happen in a few distinct pieces of the butt, so you should look around a little to discover where precisely the blockage has happened. An odd little fortuitous event is that the energy blockage is likely going to happen in a similar spot on the two cheeks, so if you discover the spot on one cheek, basically begin squeezing a similar spot on the other cheek also.

Apply a similar round movement with the tips of your fingers that you used on your partner's bosom. These energy blockages may require some more pressure, notwithstanding, so if your partner can't feel anything when you are rubbing that person, simply having a go at using your thumb.

You may confront trouble finding the pressure point right now in the body, particularly if your partner has been skilled with a breathtaking posterior. This is because the energy pathways are covered underneath a great deal of substance. Bosoms once in a while ever posture such an issue, regardless of whether the bosoms being referred to are huge.

This is because the pressure points situated in bosoms are not as profound as the ones in the rear. Henceforth, if you are confronting troublesome finding your partner's pressure point, use your thumb, and it will work. If your thumb is as yet not adequate, have a go at using something inflexible like a pen to apply pressure, simply ensure you use the backside of the pen and not the pointy end!

Using such a device will assist you with providing unimaginably engaged pressure onto the energy blockage, encouraging a speedy scattering of energy and, in the process, most likely turning your partner on a lot.

Chapter 10. What Is Kamasutra

A lot of people have heard the term (often mispronounced as Karma Sutra). However, not a lot of people really can define the term as a whole. They know that it relates to sex, but they are not sure exactly what it is that the term implies.

Well, you are right that it relates to sex, but that is not the entire truth. Kamasutra is romancing and getting intimate with your partner that reaches a realm entirely outside of sex to make sex more exciting and more intense. While the term relies heavily on sexual positions in today's age, it still revolves around the idea that humans are inherently sexual creatures and to staunch that sexuality is inhumane and cruel to our bodies. It brings sex out of the bedroom and into the rest of the world in a way that makes it feel discreet and yet oh so naughty at the same time.

If you are a shy person and feel that you would not be able to do anything sexual in public, do not worry. You are most likely not going to go for a quick shag in the park (unless that is something you are into, though you could run into some serious legal issues if you are caught). Most of the sexuality out in your public life relies on gestures and body language, minute and subtle touches, and communication to drive the mind wild. You could be preparing your partner for the bedroom, and the people around you could have no idea what you are doing or that you are even doing anything. That is the beautiful thing about Kamasutra. You can do all the dirty things you could imagine, and no one else than your partner would be the wiser.

Origin of the Term

This is an ancient Hindu term. Interesting fact. A lot of people see the Hindi people as Muslims; chaste, modest human beings who deny their sexual desires. It is quite the opposite. Hindi people are very sexual people. They embrace human nature, thinking it is a crime to do otherwise.

Take a look at the traditional clothing that women from India wear. They often keep their midriffs exposed and wear skirts that are at an angle to show more of one leg than the other. Their tops are often just high enough to keep from exposing their breasts while still allowing a little room for the imagination. They wear veils that accentuate their long hair rather than hide it. They are often adorned with jewels and other shiny objects. This is to show the natural beauty of a woman, rather than cover it up, while still keeping enough hidden to give the air of mystery and excitement. That is what Kamasutra is about. Being open with your sexual nature, but not too much so that you feel excited about the options the night can hold.

Even the men in Hindi culture dress somewhat provocatively. They often wear silk shirts that are unbuttoned at the top few buttons and loose, flowing pants that give the allusion of broadness. Their clothes are designed to allure women of their culture. Everything about the Hindi culture is beautiful, open, and gives the air of sexuality.

So it only makes sense that the term originated from one of the first cultures to embrace sexuality. It comes from the Hindi terms Kama and

Sutra. Sutra is translated to mean a line or a connection holding things together. The Kama is more in-depth than that, as it is one of the four goals in Hindi's life. It is the third goal, the goal of sexual desire and pleasure.

Outside the Sex

The original *Kama Sutra* was written sometime in the second century CE. It has since been adapted far beyond the origins to nearly become a sex manual for people who want to go the distance but are not quite sure how. However, what the newer texts fail to realize is that it goes further than sex. You need more than a manual of positions to spice up your love life because eventually, you are going to have tried all of the positions, and then you will end up back to square one.

Once you learn that it is not just about the body but also about the mind, you will find that it is a lot easier to get things going. You will see that not only has your sex life increased, and your libido will rise as well. You will want to come home to your partner and ravage their bodies, and the mental connection that you will begin to feel with them will make it even better.

So there you have it. A quick run-down of what Kamasutra is. The more you understand it, the easier it will be to master it.

Chapter 11. Benefits of Kama Sutra

Everybody understands that changing up sex positions and trying new things is good for their sex life. Even still, people choose to stick with what they are used to for one reason or the other. Let's take a moment to look at the benefits of trying new things in bed, specifically the Kama Sutra.

Different Perspective

When you change up your sex positions, you are also changing your perspective in bed. You get to see new areas of your partner's body and experience different types of stimulation.

This is a very important thing for men because their eyes are the second most important zone after his penis. Women love with their ears, but men love with their eyes. Men have visual sex, which is why they are more likely to watch porn. When they get to see something new that is also exciting, it only makes the sex that much better.

For example, in missionary, you only see each other's faces, but if you move to doggy style, he gets a perfect view of her rear. The same is true if the woman gets on top. They get a nice view of each other's chest.

Different Sensations

The penis touches a different area of the vagina and enters at varying depths. This changes how sex feels for him and her. For women, they are all different. They feel different things even if they are stimulated in the exact same spot. For men, they feel pretty much the same thing.

Boost in Confidence

Simply following the Kama Sutra can help boost a person's self-confidence. The actual Kamasutra provides tips on how to boost a person's confidence and guides you to help make your personality magnetic.

Help Women Reach an Orgasm

The worst thing for a woman is not reaching orgasm during sex. Every woman is unique in what she needs to climax, so trying out new things in bed can help her to get exactly what she wants.

Why would you risk your relationship when all you need to do is change up your positions so that she actually has an orgasm? It is important for men to understand exactly how their partner's body works so that they know what she needs.

Tone the Organism

In Eastern medicine, there is a notion that all parts of the organs and body are connected, and each part can be influenced by another part. Genitals of man and woman have many representative areas of every vital organ within the body. During sex and in various sexual positions, these parts are stimulated. This means that you can be helping other areas of your body when you are having sex.

Practical Exercises to Increase Male Orgasmic Control

Every man wants to have a more intense orgasm that lasts a long time. It is quite simple to reach an orgasm. It only takes some knowledge and patience. Sit back, relax, and read on.

Strengthening the Love Muscle

Having good looking abs might get you noticed and possibly lucky. If you would like to get the most out of your sexual experiences, you have to work on your pubococcygeal muscle. This sits on the floor of the pelvis, and it controls your urine stream and the muscle spasms when you have an orgasm. This is the reason sex therapists and doctors recommend that you strengthen it to lessen the chances of having premature ejaculations and to improve your orgasm.

Kegel exercises aren't just for females. They also strengthen the man's pelvis power. When you feel the urge to urinate, squeeze the muscle to stop the flow. When you have found this muscle, squeeze it. Now, hold this for two seconds and release. Do this exercise 20 times at least three times every day. You need to hold it for longer intervals gradually. Don't stop doing it either. Kegel exercises have to be performed regularly to help keep those muscles strong.

Edging

There isn't a technique that is as successful as strengthening a male orgasm as edging or holding back right before you orgasm. Then you rest until you have control, and them working at it again. You continue to do this until it becomes second nature.

You can practice this by masturbating until you are ready to orgasm and then stop. Get your breathing under control and wait at least 30 seconds before you continue. If this doesn't work for you, you can stop your ejaculation by squeezing the tip of the penis or gently pulling on the testicles right when you are ready to have an orgasm. Then do it all over again. Once you have mastered edging, you will be able to have dry or contractile orgasms. This gives you all the same feeling as having an orgasm but without the loss of erection. If you continue to practice this, you could even experience multiple orgasms.

Increase Testosterone Levels

Watch a big mixed martial arts match, go to the gym and workout, watch a gangster movie, go for a run. Any one of the above activities can raise your testosterone levels. Researchers have found that when a man has a lot of testosterone in his bloodstream, he will have a better chance of having an orgasm.

Stop Masturbating

I know this contradicts what was said above, but once you have learned how to "edge," you don't have to do this as often. Masturbating isn't going to give you an eye-rolling, mind-blowing orgasm. Everybody in the world knows it. The male body will release 400 percent more prolactin right after a man penetrates a vagina than it does after he masturbates. Prolactin is a male hormone that makes you feel satisfied sexually.

The evolutionary forces at play have always rewarded behaviors that are associated with reproduction. Having vaginal, penile sex is sexual behavior that gets passed down through the genes.

Deep Breathing

If you were to ask any sex therapist how to reach a full body orgasm, they would tell you that controlled breathing is the key. If you keep your breathing regular and deep, this allows for a more intense arousal to build. Your orgasm will continue to be more satisfying. Breathing too fast will increase the excitement and will push you over the edge.

Breathing can intensify the male orgasm by bringing more oxygen into the arousal process. You should take shallow breaths in through the nose and deep breaths out through the mouth to get rid of muscular and psychological tension that will help to intensify your orgasm.

Using the Brain

Orgasms are all about activating your brain. Our brains control everything and activate our genitals. Women experience a lot of activity in the brain's area that is connected to emotions, whereas a man only experiences most of their brain activity in their secondary somatosensory cortex that deals with physical sensations. The good news? To have a better orgasm, you need to have your partner focus on your penis while you focus on the sensation that you get from it.

Keep Your Feet Warm

Seriously, scientists have found that men who have cold feet have a harder time reaching orgasm than men who wear socks or have warm feet. When the man is comfortable, he will be more relaxed, and relaxation is the key to having greater orgasms. If you are afraid your woman will make fun of you in nothing but your socks, you could turn the heat up or put them in warm water before she gets there.

Chapter 12. Kama Sutra Preparation and Steps

It is important to make sure both you and your partner are ready to try some new sexual positions. Preparation is the key, and it is important to agree in advance, which you will try. The Kama Sutra is something you will need to practice and not take too seriously, especially if things don't go right!

Kama Sutra Preparation

Step 1—Make Time

Fix date in your diaries; not only does this help you make sure you make time for yourselves and your relationship, but it also builds anticipation. Together choose a position or a warmup that you feel comfortable trying.

Step 2—Create a Loving Space

Beneficial for creating the mood, set the scene. For most people, this will be the bedroom, but it could be anywhere that is safe, that you feel comfortable in, and that will offer you privacy.

To prepare the room:

- Eliminate any annoying distractions.

- Declutter.

- Redecorate if necessary.

- Enhance the room with flowers, candles, soft furnishings.

- Create an ambiance using scent, a powerful element for sensuality (try essential oils such as ylang-ylang or rose).

- Make the space as comfortable as possible, using pillows, blankets, and soft sheets.

- Play music quietly that is gentle and mood evoking, make sure it is something that both of you like.

- Turn the lights down and shut out the world.

Step 3—Set the Ambience

Have a candle-lit bath together beforehand.

Warm-up your body to help move energy, have a good shake of your legs and arms, loosen your shoulders, and roll your neck.

Kama Sutra Top Tips to Try

Keep Your Eyes Open

Making love with your eyes open is a tried and tested way to evoke deep intimacy and connection with your partner. Some people might find this difficult, so introduce in stages if need be. It is often hard to be seen when we feel at our most vulnerable but being aware of the act of love by witnessing it will make the experience far more connecting and transformative.

Make Love Slowly

Decide beforehand that you will make love slowly. The journey is more important than the destination here. Spend time arousing each other; foreplay is essential. The longer you take stimulating each other, the more the sexual energy will build. Pause if you need it. Use the time to fully connect to each other, enjoying the moment and allowing yourself to linger there. Breathe slowly, concentrating on your breath. Consciously postpone the point of reaching orgasm. When you do reach orgasm, you will find it is a much more intense and pleasurable experience. Much more stress and tension will be released, and the benefits of this both physically and mentally will last much longer.

Breathe Slowly Before the Climax

When you feel, you might climax, and you want to prolong the experience slow down your breathing. Usually, when orgasming, we breathe more quickly, particularly women. If you instead take deep, slow breaths down to your stomach, the orgasm will last much longer and be of greater intensity.

Choose the Right Positions

Remember to choose positions for sexual intercourse that won't make you reach orgasm too quickly; the slower you go, the more energy there will be, and the orgasm you and your partner will have will be far more intense and pleasurable.

Kama Sutra Kissing Techniques

There are many reasons why we kiss, and there are many types of kissing. Kissing is a forming bond action between two people. Most of us are familiar with the kiss on the cheek as a welcoming gesture, the air kiss, the kiss on the forehead as an act of affection, and so forth. There is also the kissing we share with our partner.

The Kama Sutra places significant importance on the kiss, and there are many different kisses to evoke different emotions and passion. Try kissing more before moving on to sex.

Quite often, the act of kissing leads to sexual intercourse and is an indication that we are feeling in need of close physical contact. Most of us become habitual kissers with our partners; we kiss in the same way, using the same kisses. The Kama Sutra offers a whole new perspective to the art of kissing, sharing techniques to keep things passionate and exciting.

Here are some kissing techniques from the Kama Sutra to try:

The Askew Kiss

Key words: passion, intensity.

A very simple kiss and one you are probably already familiar with doing. To do this kiss, heads are tilted in opposite directions, which allows the tongue to enter deeply; it is a fantastic kiss to provoke a profound, passionate sexual experience.

The Bent Kiss

Key words: romance, gentle, Tantric.

A romantic kissing technique. One will tilt their head back and take the chin of their partner in their hand and then kiss them gently; this is a great kiss for starting slow; it can be used in Tantric Sex too and is a real sexual energy builder.

The Direct Kiss

Key words: excitement, foreplay, passion.

The kiss is performed facing each other and involves licking, sucking, flicking of the tongue; it is playful and steamy and is a sign that a very passionate encounter will follow.

The Top Kiss

Key words: excitement, sensation, foreplay.

One partner with their teeth pulls and sucks the other partner's top lip; the other partner does the same to the other's bottom lip. Alternating this, so it is vice versa with the use of the tongue in between, can be a great passion builder and is perfect for foreplay as it excites the senses.

The Pressure Kiss

Key words: sensation, passion.

To practice this, the partner must have the mouth closed while the other bites the lips. (More nip than bite—you need to be careful that you don't cause pain!) This kiss can be adapted if you prefer not to bite, and instead, while one partner remains with lips closed, the other kisses using a lot of pressure.

The Clip Kiss

Key words: teasing, anticipation.

To do this, kiss one partner using their tongue to touch and flick and lick the other person's lips and tongue; it is very pleasurable for both.

The Throbbing Kiss

Key words: romance, tenderness, and love.

This kiss involves one partner giving the other lots of small kisses on the mouth.

Chapter 13. Flirting and Courtship

Flirting and courtship are two very important aspects of any relationship, as, without them, we would never be able to woo our partners and attract them to us. We all have our own unique style of flirting, some of us being better at it than others, but thankfully the Kama Sutra lays out exactly what we should be doing in order to be the best flirter possible.

Before we dive into the art of courtship and the tricks to up your flirting game, we will break down exactly what flirting and courtship are and how they differ. Flirting is something that is done with a less serious intention in mind than when you court someone. Flirting can be both sexual as well as friendly, and people can engage in it for fun just as much as they can use it to attract a partner. Typically flirting involves using both verbal and non-verbal communication in order to let someone know that you are interested in them. It can involve a wink, touching someone's arm, laughing at their jokes, or any other ways in which you showcase your interest.

Courting, on the other hand, is more serious in nature, and it is dating someone with the intention of marrying them. Some religious beliefs feel that the only acceptable form of dating is courting, while others engage in courting, not for religious reasons but because they are simply at a point in life where they are looking to get married. Courting can, and should, involve flirting, but it is used to win the other person over and entice them to want to marry you. It is never simply used to instigate a fling or sexual encounter, as that would be in direct contradiction to the point of courting.

Now that we have a basic understanding of the two terms, what exactly does the Kama Sutra say when it comes to courting and flirting?

Meeting the Person You Want to Date

To begin with, the Kama Sutra starts by mentioning that anyone looking to court another should be realistic in their approach. What this means is that any quality that they are seeking in another, they should possess that quality themselves; otherwise, they have no right to expect it of their partner. For instance, if you want your partner to be extremely good looking, you should also be extremely good looking; otherwise, you should not put such a demand on someone else. Once you have your expectations in check, then you can begin the process of searching for your partner.

So, how does one go about seeking out a woman in ancient times when there was no social media and no dating apps? Well, the Kama Sutra suggests the following ways:

- A woman who is ready to be married should be dressed up nicely by her family and placed in a location where she can be seen.

- Women seeking a husband should attend events such as sporting matches and marriage ceremonies.

- Men should throw parties in which games are played, causing everyone to interact with each other.

- Through friendships, two people can then meet and get to know each other.

- By asking their parents, a man can have a wife arranged for him.

Of course, we can add much more to this list for current times, so if you are at the point in your life where you are looking to meet someone and build towards marriage, or a future in general, you can try the following more common suggestions as well:

- **Try going online and joining a dating site**—Nowadays, there are numerous different sites, all catering to different individuals and desires, so you are likely to find a site that is perfect for you and finding a partner that matches what you are after.

- **Ask your friends to hook you up with someone**—We know the idea of going on a blind date sounds terrifying, but your friends do know you well, so there is always the chance that they might know someone who fits in with what you are looking for.

- **Participate in a sport or hobby**—Take up a new activity that interests you in order to meet new people and also meet someone who shares similar interests with you. Not only will you already have something to talk about, but it gets you out of the house and on a mini-date right from day one.

- **Take the bus to work**—While your morning commute is never fun, why not turn it into an opportunity to meet someone? Public transportation puts you in close proximity to new people that you have never met before.

However, you choose to approach meeting someone, that is only the first step in courtship, as the real work is what comes afterward.

Beginning a Courtship

Once you have found an individual who interests you, who you would like to get closer with, and possibly start a relationship, how are you supposed to let them know that you are interested? In modern times, we have many ways of determining if someone is interested in us, and many of these various ways fall under the heading of flirting. When we are attracted to someone, either physically or mentally, or both, our bodies automatically respond to them in specific ways. Some of what we do is deliberate, while other actions are completely subconscious and are naturally done simply because we want to be near someone.

Some of the common ways of flirting that you may be more familiar with are:

- Making direct eye contact.

- Holding eye contact longer than normal.

- Smiling when you look at a person.

- Touching them on the arm when you talk.

- Winking from across a room.

- Complimenting the other person.

- Biting of the lip.

- Playing with your hair.

- Mirroring another person's movements.

- Laugh at their silly jokes.

- Stand closely.

- Stare at their lips.

- Keep your arms uncrossed and open.

- Tease them playfully.

- Drop a witty pick-up line.

- Send a flirtatious text message.

Sadly, you won't find any of these located within the Kama Sutra, as back in ancient India, flirting and courting were done much differently. To compare with the above list, let's take a look at different ways in which the Kama Sutra suggests a man flirts with a woman to show her that he is interested and to engage her attention:

- Spend time with her and entertain her with games.

- Pick flowers and turn them into a garland.

- Cook meals together.

- Play with dice or cards.

- Playgroup games such as hide and seek.

- Do gymnastic exercises together.

- Show kindness to her friends.

- Partake in services for her maid's daughter to win her over.

- Get her gifts that no other girls have.

- Give her handmade dolls and wooden figures.

- Create temples for her dedicated to different goddesses.

- Make her see him as someone who can do everything for her.

- Meet her in private.

- Tell her exciting stories.

- Perform tricks and juggle.

- Sing for her and take her to festivals.

- Give her flowers and jewelry.

- Teach her nurse's daughter the 64 forms of pleasure.

While many of these sound a bit strange in today's time, there is a lot we can take away from this list. Mainly, everything described above is meant to make the man stand out from other men that may have an interest in the same woman. This is exactly what modern-day flirting and courting involves as well, as you want to make the other person see what you have to offer and what they will find in you that they cannot find in someone else. Flirting and courting are meant to entice another person, that is their sole purpose, and to let that person know that you would like to be in a relationship with them, or at the very least engage in some sort of romantic endeavor.

Many people get stressed out by the idea of flirting, and so often, you will hear individuals remark that they are unable to flirt or are the worst at doing so. This is simply a false idea that they have gotten into them here, and they are making it into something much more complicated than it needs to be. Flirting does not need to be anything more than smiling at a person you like or going out of your way to do something nice for them. All you are aiming to do is make them feel special and noticed, and to hopefully get them to notice you in return. The best way to go about it if you lack confidence is to simply start off small. You don't need to perform a magic trick or juggle, and instead, you can simply compliment their outfit or send them a text asking about their day. The basic act of taking notice goes a very long way as it shows the person you are thinking of them and that you are interested in who they are. Don't overcomplicate things, and let it progress naturally as you feel more comfortable. Once you get outside of your own head, you will find flirting to be one of the most natural acts possible.

A Woman's State of Mind

Within the Kama Sutra, Vatsyayana goes into detail about a woman's state of mind during flirting and courtship and breaks down the different ways she may feel and react, as well as how many should respond to her. Some of the advice is practical and useful even in today's world, but other tips are much more non-consensual and should not ever be utilized. Here are the mindsets that are mentioned, along with the details attributed to each one:

A Woman Who Listens but Does Not Show Any Interest

In this scenario, a man should attempt to persuade her by using a middle man instead of just doing it on his own. A good option would be her nurse's daughter or one of her friends.

If a Woman Meets a Man Once and Then the Next Time Is Better Dressed

This indicates that she is very interested, and thus the man will need to do little in order to win her over. If, however, after a long period of time, she still does not consent to be with him, then he should be wary but still keep her as a close friend.

When a Woman Avoids a Man Out of Respect

In this scenario, it will be difficult to win her over, but the man can do so by keeping her as a close friend and also employing the assistance of a very crafty middle man.

If a Woman Turns a Man Down Harshly

When this happens, a man should abandon his attempts to win her over and move on to someone else, for she had no interest in anything he has to offer her.

When Meeting Privately, She Allows His Touch but Pretends Not to Notice

If this happens, then it means she is interested but playing coy, so he should continue on with his advances. It will require extra patience, but he can begin by putting his arm around her while she sleeps and seeing how she reacts. If it is a favorable reaction, then he can continue on by drawing her closer to him and continuing on from there.

Chapter 14. Emotional and Physical Intimacy

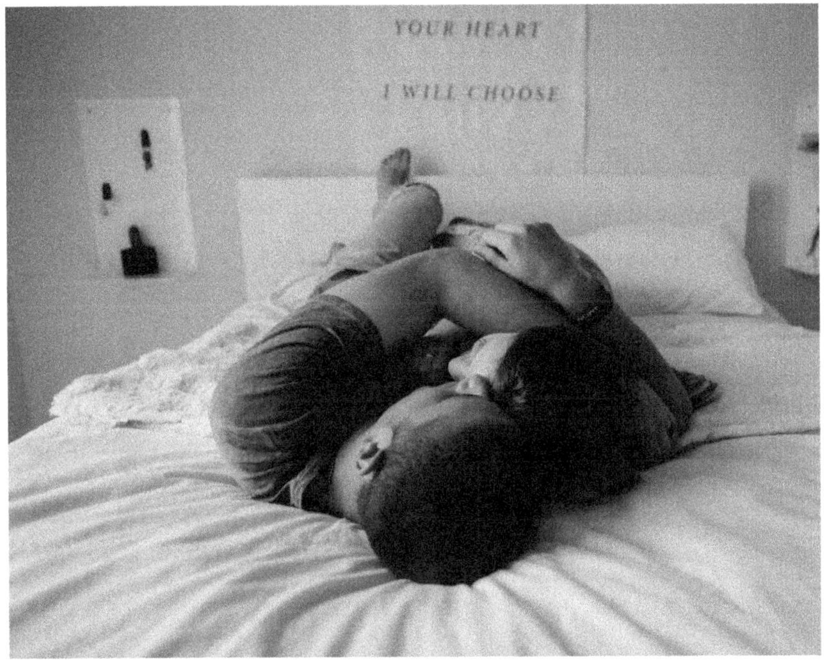

Intimacy, in a general sense, is defined as mutual openness and vulnerability. There are different ways that intimacy can show up in a relationship, as long as it involves giving and receiving vulnerability. There are different, more specific types of intimacy that are present in different relationships. In this part, we will focus on two of these forms of intimacy—emotional intimacy and physical intimacy.

Emotional vs. Physical Intimacy

In this part, I am going to define emotional and physical intimacy before comparing the two in a variety of ways.

Emotional intimacy is the ability to express oneself in a mature and open manner, which leads to a deep emotional connection between two people. Saying things like "I love you" or "you are very important to me" are examples of this. It is also the ability to respond in a mature and open way when someone expresses themselves to you by saying things like "I'm sorry" or "I love you too." This type of intimacy is found in romantic relationships and in some friendships or familial relationships.

Physical intimacy is the type of intimacy that most people think of when they hear the term, and it is the kind that we have been addressing. This is the type of intimacy that includes physical touch, including sex, and all activities related to sex. However, it also involves other non-sexual types of physical contact, such as hugging and kissing.

How to Increase Intimacy

In a romantic or sexual relationship, intimacy is a given. You would not enter a romantic relationship without some degree of emotional intimacy, and a sexual relationship, by definition, involves physical intimacy. For a romantic relationship to be successful, both forms of intimacy must be present between the partners. Without intimacy, there is nothing that sets a romantic relationship apart from an everyday friendship. Intimacy is something that must be worked at and maintained consistently, especially emotional intimacy. In a romantic relationship, however, physical intimacy must be maintained as well, as this is one way of showing the other person that you feel strongly for them. If intimacy is lacking or if it fades over time, there are some things that you can do to revive or rekindle it.

The first way to restore intimacy in a relationship or to develop it in the first place is through communication. Communication is key in a relationship of any sort, but especially in a romantic relationship. Communicating is the only sure way to know where the other person stands in terms of their thoughts and feelings. Being able to be vulnerable and open with your emotions is a requirement for intimacy. It is necessary to share oneself with the other person in a relationship. This mutual sharing of yourselves is what will lead to intimacy in the first place or an increase in intimacy.

It is important to communicate about your needs for intimacy on a recurring basis since people will grow and change over the course of a relationship. Especially in a long-term relationship, being aware of when a person's intimacy needs change is important to maintaining a good level of intimacy.

When working on intimacy, it is helpful to start slow by talking about things that are easier for you to open up about—like your future goals or your ideal job. This is still a way to open up without pushing yourself too far right away. It can be scary to be that vulnerable with someone. It is also helpful to note that for many people, there are things that they consciously avoid thinking about, as they may be painful to address. It will be very difficult for them to voice these things to themselves, so allow them to start slowly, and don't be offended if you feel like there are topics that they are uncomfortable talking about.

Many people have a fear of intimacy, and this is also worth noting. Because intimacy needs trust in order to develop, it can be hard for some people who have had past experiences that make it hard for them to trust people. By being aware of this, it may help you to understand why your partner has trouble opening up. It may also help you if you have a fear of intimacy as you can explain this to your partner in order to ask for the patience you will need as you begin to open up and be vulnerable with them.

When it comes to improving intimacy, it is a slow build and not a race to the finish line. Be patient with yourself and your partner, and try to see intimacy as a growing experience between you that will continue throughout the entire duration of your relationship.

Best Positions for Intimacy

As I mentioned, intimacy is something that needs to be worked at and practiced. It is something that needs to be actively maintained and does not stay as is when achieved once. As a couple, there are many ways to work on your intimacy, and sex is one of those ways. Sex also happens to come with many other benefits, but these positions we will explore now are chosen because they are the best for creating intimacy and connection for you and your partner.

The Lotus

Arguably the most intimate position of them all is The Lotus. The Lotus position is most intimate because of the closeness of your entire bodies, infinitely pressed against each other at all points from head to toe while being face to face.

The man sits on the bed cross-legged, his torso upright. His penis is erect and ready to get it on. The woman climbs on top of him and sits in his lap, wrapping her arms and legs around him. He holds her by wrapping his arms around her as well. With some shifting, they slide his penis inside of her. In this position, both people will be grinding more than they will be thrusting or humping. This is also what makes it so intimate. Grinding face to face while she is sitting on his lap with him inside of her, that is about as intimate as it gets.

In this position, you will not be doing any crazy thrusting, so it is ideal for a steamy make-out session, as your mouths will be so close that you can feel each other's breath the entire time. You can look into each other's eyes and whisper sweet nothings to them as you share this intimate experience.

Slow Grind

Another position that makes for a high level of intimacy and closeness is the Slow Grind position. In this position, the man sits down with his legs extended and leans back on his hands. The woman climbs on top of him, facing him, and puts his penis inside of her. she extends her legs past him and leans back on her hands as well. In this position, they cannot move too much without risking his penis sliding out of her, so they are restricted to a slow grind. They both slowly grind their hips into each other and move gently. With both of their arms occupied to hold them up, they can only move their hips, and this makes for an intimate mood with no distractions of arms and legs moving about. They are seated facing each other as well, so they will look at each other in the eyes as they slowly grind and pleasure each other. You can see why this position is such an intimate one for a couple to try together.

Chapter 15. Embraces

A large part of Kama Sutra techniques revolves around foreplay and getting the body ready for the pleasure that is to come. There are few actions that are as stimulating as an embrace, where two bodies come together, feeding off each other's warmth and experiencing the different textures and contours. The embrace is also referred to as "Chatushshashti." You need to be able to explore the body of your lover so that you find those delicate areas and hot spots which will heighten the pleasure,

The typical embrace will mean that you are using more than just your arms. In Kama Sutra, you need to embrace using your entire body—a far cry from a hug. Starting at the top and moving down to the bottom of your feet, let your entire body come into contact with that of your lover, using smooth and circular movements that can best be described as a gentle caress. Alternate the pressure by touching some areas lightly and rubbing other areas with more intensity. You know the body of your lover, so by their reactions, you will figure out which are the areas that you need to place your focus on. There is no right or wrong way to carry out an embrace, so you can choose to do it standing up, or you could lie down and embrace while you are on the bed.

When you are embracing, remember that there is more to your body than just your hands. Use your hands as little as possible and instead take advantage of your cheeks and chest, your shoulders, and even your thighs. The embrace should have a gentle rubbing of your entire body for total stimulation. Also, your lips are a secret weapon, and you can kiss your lover gently, almost like you would imagine the flutter of a butterfly. The key is to make the process of embracing slowly and sensually.

Not all the embraces are considered equal in Kama Sutra, as each one can bring out different feelings and pleasures. There are twelve in total, most of which you typically carry out naturally. Here are the embraces for you to try as part of your foreplay.

The Touching Embrace

This embrace normally takes place even before you have taken the time to set the mood and create a room that is designed to elevate your sensuality. This embrace is often unexpected, a soft touch that a man gives a woman to get her attention. There is so much a woman can read from this touch, as it can communicate affection, desire, love, and lust. To prepare your partner for the final act of making love and intercourse, you should give them light touches for the entire day. This will have their minds racing, thinking about all the fantastic things that are to come. This is one of the first embraces that are ever done, typically before a couple has ever engaged in sexual intercourse.

The Forehead Embrace

This is an embrace that is all about the intensity of feeling and the gentleness of a budding relationship. One of the lovers will use their mouths to plant gentle and light kisses on the others' eyelids, mouth, and forehead. This embrace ensures that there is close contact between the two lovers and that they have the chance to look deep into each other's eyes from close range. It signifies the growth of a relationship and that there are deeply caring and affection. The gentle nature of this embrace can quickly stimulate a lover.

The Rubbing Embrace

This is an embrace that is done when two lovers have the opportunity to get close together when they are in a public place, which happens to be a little lonely. Usually, they would be walking together with their hands intertwined, and when they find a place where there is no one about, they will take the chance to rub their bodies against one another. This ensures that they can feel each other's contours and helps with their closeness as they look forward to going indoors and finding other ways that they can get close to each other.

The Twining of a Creeper

An embrace that is typically done by women; this embrace calls for the woman to wrap herself around the man and cling to him using her arms and her legs. Their heads are bent towards each other as though they are about to kiss—but they do not. It is all about closeness and communicating love and possession through touch. There is also a sound that should be made with this embrace; the woman should gently say the words out "sut sut", as they have a way of increasing the intensity of the embrace. This embrace embodies affection and is deeply personal.

The Climbing Embrace

This is also referred to as the "vrikshadhirudhaka." Here is another embrace where the woman uses her legs to go around the body of the man. In this embrace, she will have one foot that is placed on her lover's foot, while her other foot is placed upon his thighs. To ensure she is balanced, one of her arms will go around the back of the man, and the other arm shall hold on to the man's shoulders. While in this embrace, the woman will make some sounds that are similar to singing, or she will make a gentle cooing noise. She is supposed to appear as if she is reaching up to his face so that she can give him a kiss. It is the reaching upwards that gives this embrace its name.

The Pressing Embrace

Have you ever watched a love scene when one of the lovers gets pressed up against a wall, while the other users their body to press against them? This action is highly stimulating, as you feel the contours of your lover's body against yours, and often, can feel their heart racing on your chest. The pressing embrace is typically an embrace where you press your entire body against your partner, like a hug but with more intensity. This is a brilliant way for you to communicate the passion that you are feeling and also to bring out the natural excitement in your bodies.

The Piercing Embrace

This is an embrace that is meant to tantalize a man, giving him a sample of what he can expect later during a period of lovemaking. For this embrace, a woman will find a quiet place where she is able to work on getting the full attention of the man. She will then bend forward before him as if she is reaching to pick up something from the ground. While she is in this position, she will use her breasts and her nipples to "pierce" a man by making a gentle movement that rubs against him. The main is them meant to take hold of the breasts and gently fondle them. This is an embrace that is done before two people have become fully comfortable with each other.

The Milk and Water Embrace

This embrace is also referred to as "kshiraniraka." During foreplay, things can get so intense that you want to feel your partner inside of you if you are a woman, or you want penetration if you are a man. In the midst of all your kissing, you get into a position where you could experience intercourse, but your clothes are creating a barrier that stops it from happening. As your sexual organs rub against each other, you are stimulated but have not yet given in to the temptation to start full intercourse. At this point, the foreplay has taken a turn that is highly erotic, and the embrace is highly passionate. In this embrace, the woman will typically be sitting on the man's lap, or they could be lying in bed with bodies rubbing against each other. It is meant to resemble a mixture of milk and water.

The Jaghana Embrace

To do this embrace, you need to first identify the Jaghana. This is an area that can be found between the belly button and the thighs of a woman. To stimulate the woman during foreplay, this embrace requires the man to press this area using his own body, as though he is in a mounting motion. Then, he should gently scratch or bite her while using his hands to hold onto her neck or her hair. The pain that results from this embrace should be very light and gentle, and this changes the pace of the entire period of foreplay, making it highly sensual. Gentle scratches along the back and arms are very erotic, and as long as there is no aggression, this can be the final embrace before moving into full intercourse.

The Sesamum Seed With Rice Embrace

This occurs when the woman and the man are lying together on a bed. They use their arms and legs to hold onto each other as tightly as possible by ensuring that they are fully encircled. While they are in this embrace, their bodies shall rub together so that they can feel the strength of their arousal. This is an intense embrace, which is often done at the end of the penetrative intercourse to reinforce the feeling of closeness in the afterglow.

The Thigh Embrace

This is an embrace that begins with a lack of consent and ends with a transfer of power that is electric and stimulating. A man or a woman will be lying down on the bed, and one of them shall forcibly press a thigh or both their thighs of their lover in between their own. Then they shall hold the position so that their genitals are rubbing against the leg of their partners.

The Breast Embrace

This is an embrace that brings together the breasts of both the man and the woman. In this embrace, the man will bring his breasts and then place them in between the breasts belonging to the woman that he wants to make love to. After he has placed it, he will press down on her, effectively rubbing against her to bring her stimulation to its peak.

Embraces often come quite naturally when you are looking for closeness for your partner, so although these embraces are considered to be essential for Kama Sutra, that should not stop you from having any other embraces which are natural to you. All that is important at the end of it is that there is passion in the embrace so that the resulting intercourse can be fruitful.

Chapter 16. Kama Sutra and Oral Sex

In the original ancient text of the Kama Sutra, oral sex had a significant role to play. It was essential to stimulate and around a lover as much as possible before actual penetration would take place. Oral sex makes it possible to reach orgasm in a powerful way, such that the body experiences tremors, and intercourse becomes all the more fulfilling. It was also meant to be given to both the woman and the man, slowly and purposefully.

Licking of the Rose Petals

The term that is used to describe the act of cunnilingus is known as licking of the rose petals, and there were several techniques that can be applied for intense arousal and orgasm. The first of these is known as the quivering kiss. This technique makes use of both the fingers and the tongue to drive one to intense pleasure. To begin, the man would gently take hold of the lips of the vagina and then ever so slowly pinch them together so that the entry into the vagina can be tightened. Using his lips, he would place soft kisses on them, in the same way as though he was kissing the lips that are on her face. This would bring them to a new level of intimacy, revealing gentle and tender care and love.

From this technique, the man would move to the next step into what is known as the circling tongue. Here, the lips of the vagina would then be opened and spread using the fingers, allowing the tongue to gently enter the walls of the vagina. While the tongue goes in and out slowly, the rest of his face would be circling in the area so that the lips and the chin make contact with the clitoris. This technique is also given the name "jihvabhramanaka."

The next technique is known as the tongue massage. This is the term that is used to describe the thrusting of the tongue in and out of the vagina. The man has to build up to an intense rhythm that leaves the woman curling her toes in pleasure. Using the tongue, the man should massage the entire area in and around the vagina instead of placing focus on one specific place. In addition, the pressure of each thrust should be varied to add to the element of surprise and also to ensure that the act does not become boring for the woman.

From this point, the focus can shift to the clitoris in a technique that is translated to the word sucked or which is known as "chushita." This requires the man to such deeply on the lips of the vagina and then gently nibble on these lips. From here, he should move his mouth so that it is over her clitoris, and with significant pressure, suck on the clitoris to help the woman reach her orgasm. It is this small bit of flesh that has the power to drive a woman to intense heights of pleasure by instantly increasing her arousal. To add on to the sucking motion, the man should also vary the speed with which the sucking is done and vary the movement by going in circles.

To reach deeper levels, the buttocks of the woman should be cupped into the hands of the man, and the tongue should then be used to travel from the walls of the vagina up to the navel and then back down again in a movement that is called sucked up or "uchchushita." The key to ensuring maximum stimulation is to use circular movements and to vary the time that is spent between the vagina lips and the navel.

The next technique is known as stirring, and here, attention is paid to the thighs as well as to the vagina. By focusing on the highest point of the thighs, where her legs meet her buttocks, it is possible to reach a peak of stimulation. The woman needs to help by holding her thighs apart so that the tongue has better access to her sacred area, in a technique that is also referred to as "Kshobhaka." By holding and opening the thighs, the woman is sharing in the moment of pleasure by helping her partner to get better access to her inner areas.

While most of these techniques need to be done while lying down on a bed, this next technique can be done on a table. In Kama Sutra, the acts of sex and foreplay are not restricted to the bedroom as they often are in modern times. Lovers were able to explore the joys of sex in every room within their homes, and this was one way to build up anticipation and try out new techniques. "Bahuchushita," which translates to sucking hard, called for the woman to be seated on a couch, placing her feet on top of the shoulders of the man. With her balancing in this way, the man would then hold on to her waist and begin to suck on her clitoris with intensity. To relive the mounting pleasure and arousal, he also uses his tongue to lick around the entire area until she reaches her orgasm.

Sucking a Mango Fruit

For men engaging in Kama Sutra, fellatio is also known as sucking the mango fruit. This description is meant to indicate the smoothness of the fruit and the sweet juiciness of it. Even the words that are used to describe this act are sensual, mysterious, and interesting. There are also several methods that a woman can try so that she is able to please her partner.

To begin with, there is touching, which involves the use of both the hands and the mouth. This is how all fellatio techniques should start. The woman will use both of her hands to hold on to the penis and then by opening her mouth, and she will gently use her lips to kiss the tip and also just move over it, gently making small circles with her face. This ensures that there is stimulation on the most sensitive part of the penis in the technique that is also referred to as "Nimitta."

From here, one makes the next move called nominal congress. Without giving up the use of the hands, the penis is held gently, and she uses her mouth to move it around between her lips. This reaches more parts of the penis than the Nimitta but still leaves a considerable amount to be explored. This part of the process is simple to awaken the penis so that it is as hard and ready for penetration as possible. However, there is more room for deep stimulation with the next technique.

In this technique, the woman shall hold on to the penis using her hands, paying special attention to the head, which she will hold firmly. Her lips will then move up and down the shaft, from one side all the way to the other, and she will gently allow her teeth to rub against the skin on occasion. The penis is sensitive, so using the teeth excessively can kill the romance. This process is known as "Parshvatoddashta."

The next technique makes use of any foreskin that could be on the penis. The woman will hold the penis in her mouth, making sure that most of the contact is with her lips. In a technique called "Bahiha samdansha" or the outer pincers, she will slowly and gently pull back the soft foreskin and place the penis in her mouth where she uses her lips to apply pressure while she gently kisses it, making sure to use slow motion.

This is followed by the "Antaha samdansha," which is also known as the inner pincers. It is this part of stimulation that the man looks forward to the most. Here, the woman will finally slide the entire penis into her mouth, making sure that the whole process is slow and steady. She will then move her head up and down, ensuring that each time she goes up, she pulls away from a little and removes her mouth before returning it and moving back down the shaft. The end result should be rhythmic, and the warmth of her tongue and moisture from the saliva adds to the overall velvet sensual feel.

The next technique is similar to what she would do if she was kissing a man on the lips. To stop if, from movement, the woman will hold the penis in her hands and then make the O shape with her lips so that they are round. She will then place quick high pressured kisses all around the length of the penis, and amidst these kisses, she will ensure that she also sucks on the shaft. This exploration ensures that the entire penis receives some attention, which can be so stimulating that the mind of her lover goes blank from the pleasure.

The following technique is all about the tongue and how it can be best used for oral sex. In a technique that is known as "Parimrshtaka," the tongue is used to quickly flick all over and around the erect penis, and the tongue shall also make repeated strikes on the highly sensitive glans tip. One must be careful to read the body language of their lover to ensure that this action is not done so aggressively that it results in pain.

Then the "Amrachushita," or the sucking of the mango fruit, is the next technique, and the one that this Kama Sutra fellatio is named after. It is assumed at this time that the lovers are in the throes of passion and are looking for one of two results—heightened stimulation to help get ready for the penetration or the need to reach an orgasm. The woman should take in as much of the penis as she can in her mouth without choking and, with wild abandon, suck hard on it, being sure to move her head up and down while doing so. The technique is meant to resemble what a person would be doing to a mango when trying to rid it of all the fruit.

Finally, the fellatio is finished with "Sangara," an act that is so intimate it may drive a man to the edge of his desire. Here, the woman senses that the man is close to orgasm. This is basically because there is a change in his breathing or movement or tension in his muscles. At this point, she ensures that the entire penis is inside her mouth and that she is sucking on it as hard as possible. In addition, there is more stimulation from the movement of her tongue, as well as her lips. While doing this, the man will become more and more aroused until finally, he releases his sperm.

With his penis still inside her mouth, the woman swallows his nectar, which is an indication that they are both highly intimate and have enjoyed the experience of oral sex.

The final method for oral stimulation is known as the crow, and it enables both the man and the woman to stimulate each other simultaneously. In modern times it is often referred to as the 69 positions. The lovers lie down on their sides, with their faces in the opposite direction.

Chapter 17. How to Last Longer

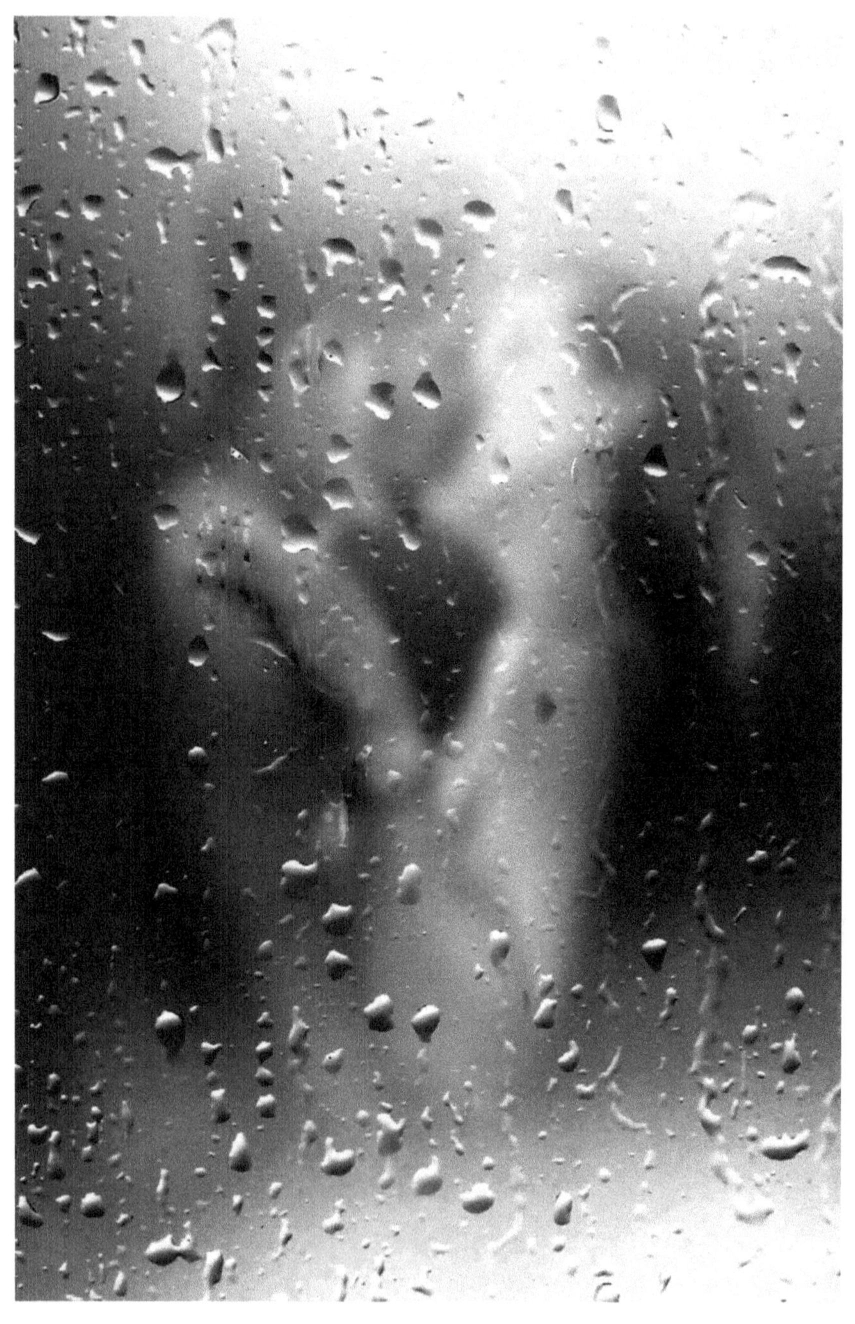

There are many theories regarding how to last longer and how to stay harder, and we will look at a few of the most effective ones now in this section. In order for both men and women to get the most out of sex and the most enjoyable orgasms, it comes down to the man's ability to last during sex. If the time it takes a man to orgasm is quite short, then the pair will have to wait until his refractory period is over before he will be able to have an erection again. During this time, the woman will still be able to be aroused and have an orgasm, but penetrative sex will not be possible. Thus, in order to have the most pleasurable and (and also more intense) orgasms and sexual encounters, I will now present some tips and tricks that the man can use to last longer in bed.

Edging

Edging is a technique that a man can use to hold off an orgasm to make himself last longer and therefore keep his erection for longer. In order to do this, he must be aware of his body and be in touch with the different feelings it has. This is similar to what we discussed earlier when talking about mindfulness and how it relates to sex.

When the man reaches a point where he is getting very close to orgasm, he will stop, or the woman will stop whatever they are doing, and he will have to take a deep breath, compose himself and hold off his orgasm. Holding back will give him time to cool down a little and come back from the edge of orgasm. During this time, while he is cooling off, he can continue to touch the woman, or the woman can touch him in other places, as long as it doesn't make him orgasm. When he is ready and has successfully held off his orgasm, they can then continue with whatever sexual acts they were doing before. Then, when he reaches the point where he is about to orgasm again, he will have to hold off once again. This can continue as many times as he can until finally, one time, he will let himself reach orgasm, and it will be much stronger and much more intense than if he had just let himself reach orgasm the first time.

This may be difficult to accomplish the first number of times because it can be hard to hold off an orgasm when you are very close. It will take practice to be able to do this technique, and especially to be able to do it multiple times over in one session. The man will have to communicate with his partner so that she knows not to keep stimulating him to the point of orgasm, especially if she was giving him oral or something of the sort.

Going to the Gym

Another way that a man can increase his endurance sexually is by going to the gym. Physical fitness is strongly related to sexual performance and endurance, so getting to the gym at least a few times a week will help him to last longer in bed, keep his erection longer, and even to be able to thrust for longer because of the cardiovascular aspect that penetrative sex comes with. This will be beneficial for both of you.

Chapter 18. Erogenous Zones

If you've watched the hit television show *Friends*, you'll remember that there are 7 erogenous zones in the female body. However, there are those who believe that there is so much more than that. In this chapter, you'll find out the obvious and less obvious erogenous zones for the male and female.

Erogenous Zones of Women

Lips

The lips are super sensitive—which is why an excellent kiss can really coax couples into full-blown sex. Containing lots of nerve endings, guys are advised to pay particular attention to the plump portions of the lips, either by biting, suckling, or nibbling.

Ears

Ears are highly sensitive—even just a whisper of wind can really get a girl's attention. Stimulate the ears by biting, nibbling, licking, and blowing into the ears. A particular technique for this body type is by exposing it to a shift of hot and cold. Play with the heat by putting the ears in your mouth and then blowing it cool.

Neck/Nape

The neck is particularly sensitive, especially the part where the shoulder meets the neck. That small shallow part is full of nerve endings and offers a thrill of pleasure for women when touched, kissed, sucked, or licked. The back of the neck is another hotspot for touch—especially low-pressure touches. This is why it's one of the most common spots touched during flirtation.

Breasts and Nipples

The breast and nipples are fairly obvious erogenous zones, but a lot of guys handle them the wrong way. Remember that breasts aren't pizza dough that needs to be worked into shape. You need to massage them slowly, starting gently before moving on to rougher handling. The underside of the breast contains some of the thinnest and, therefore, most sensitive skin, so a light touch on this area will definitely produce some results.

The nipples must be laved slowly and not sucked into the mouth quickly. Use the tip of the tongue to trace the rim of the nipples before putting the whole thing in your mouth. You'll notice that the breasts are already sensitized when the nipple turns into a pointed tip, extending outwards with the full surface ready to be kissed and touched.

Some women like teeth play when it comes to breasts since pain can be an excellent stimulant. However, try not to bite into it too much and watch out for her reaction to the bites.

Vibration also plays a huge role in the stimulation process, so try flicking your tongue back and forth over the nipples in rapid succession. Humming while keeping the nipples in your mouth can also get a girl really hot.

Lower Back

Massaging the lower back plays a huge role in getting women relaxed and therefore enhancing sexual arousal. This is excellent foreplay, and if you're thinking about going doggy style, there's nothing like a sensual touch and kiss massage on the lower back to get a girl ready. Look for the twin dimples on the lower back and concentrate most of your attention on this area. By doing this, you're increasing blood flow to the pelvis, therefore making the vagina and clitoris nerves more sensitive to the touch. This boosts pleasure upon entry and makes it easier for the girl to reach orgasm.

Vagina and Clitoris

The vagina and clitoris are obvious pleasure points but again, very few men give them the attention and stimulation that they deserve. They play a primary role in sex.

Inner Thighs

The skin of the inner thighs is especially sensitive to light touches, mainly due to the thin skin along this area. If you have a beard—bonus plus points in sensation when grazing the inner thigh! Make sure to give this body part particular attention by nuzzling and kissing the area.

Feet

The feet are always a hot zone for women—provided that you don't go overboard. A thorough massage will definitely put her in an amorous mood—especially since the feet take a LOT of abuse daily. Imagine having to wear 3-inch heels on a daily basis and see if you don't feel like your toes are going to fall off. This is why showing some love for the female feet definitely turns on the girl—and don't forget that there are lots of nerves located on foot. The arch and the little toe definitely beg attention and will get you lots of points.

Erogenous Zones of Men

For the most part, the female erogenous zones are the same as men. Note, though, that since guys have two layers of skin, they require more pressure to be felt. In this portion of the book, however, we'll pay special attention to male erogenous zones that haven't been specially mentioned in the female part.

Nipples

Male nipples deserve as much attention as female nipples, even though they don't really serve any purpose. Every bit as sensitive, you (the ladies) should treat the male nipple to some hand and oral play, mimicking exactly how you like your own nipples to be played with. This involves sucking, licking, flicking, and even biting, depending on the response of the male.

Penis

Scrotum

The scrotum is essentially the balls and is home to some of the most prominent nerve endings, which means that it can be very responsive to touch. The scrotum is both soft and firm and, for most males—requires very careful handling on the part of the female. A light massage is usually the best way to stimulate the scrotum, followed by oral sex that encompasses the balls. During blow jobs, a lot of guys find it more arousing to have the balls caressed. Prior to ejaculation, the balls tend to grow tight and retract as they prepare for release. Massaging the balls during ejaculation allows for stronger orgasms and larger amounts of semen coming out.

Perineum

This is a male-exclusive erogenous zone, although some women find this part of the body an excellent turn on as well. The perineum is that bit of skin you can find between the scrotum and the anus. This is where most of the perineal nerves are located, a portion which primarily deals with sensations of pleasure moving from the brain to the genitals and vice versa. Hence, massaging this area will really get a guy going. Best touched during a blow job, applying light and grazing pressure to this body area will give your man the kind of orgasms he's never had before.

Chapter 19. Slowing Down to Amplify Pleasure and Longevity

For those who want to last longer in bed and deliver more pleasure to your partner during your sexual experience, it should come as no surprise that slowing things way down is one of the simplest ways to achieve this end. Very often, we treat sex as an afterthought. If we have time, we might squeeze it into our days somewhere, or perhaps before bed, if we're not too tired. With this mentality, sex is only a rare treat, or perhaps a chore to be endured, rather than a major avenue of bonding and experiencing transcendental pleasure with your partner.

The health of one's relationship is every bit as important in one's life as one's physical, mental, and emotional health. When our love lives are not in harmony, it throws everything else out of whack, too. A peaceful and loving relationship, on the other hand, can bring harmony and healing when all else has gone awry.

Because our relationships are such a central part of our lives, we owe it to ourselves and our partners to treat them as a priority rather than an afterthought. One of the great insights about life is knowing that we have time for what we make time for. Give yourself permission to slow down, knowing that you and your partner deserve the fullest and most pleasure-packed experience that is possible for you.

Extending Foreplay and Slowing Sex

Our culture has groomed us to be extremely goal-oriented in our sex. The quest for the big "O" has captured our imaginations and provided content for dozens of self-help books, blogs, and advice magazines. But what if the constant striving for orgasm is all wrong?

Have you ever spent days searching for something that you lost? You scoured all the rooms in your house, picked over every inch of your car, retraced all your steps, and asked everyone you knew who may have seen the lost item. But all this was to no avail. No matter how much time you spent searching and how close to the madness you drove yourself looking for this thing, it stayed lost. Finally, you accepted defeat and moved on, almost forgetting about the item entirely… until one day when, as you were looking for something else, or perhaps not even looking at all, the long-lost item finally reappears.

Transcendental orgasms can be as elusive as the things we lose. The harder we strive for them, the less luck we will have in reaching them. When we allow ourselves to slow down and stop looking, however, this is precisely the time when we find exactly what we've been wanting.

Extending foreplay is very easy to do. The only limitation is your own imagination. Your foreplay can be as sensual, as erotic, or as playful as you wish (though the best foreplay often embodies all of these elements).

Slowing down, sex means literally that—slow down your movements. Fast and rough sex can feel amazing, but it is precisely the fastness of sexual movements that lead to quick orgasms. Our bodies can only handle so much stimulation before they need to give in. This doesn't mean that you need to do away with fast and rough sexual movements entirely; it simply means to introduce more slow and deliberate movements into the mix.

Slow down the moment of initial penetration entirely, taking the time to look deeply into your partner's eyes and savor every ounce of sensation that comes from your first pairing. You will find that the emotional feelings that wash over you with this change are every bit as intense as the physical sensations.

Once you are connected, use slow and sensual movements throughout your lovemaking. Embrace your partner, caress their face and body, run your fingers up and down their back, kiss their neck and shoulders. Engage the whole body in the lovemaking process. If you feel the urge to climax before you are both ready, stop, and take a few deep breaths until the urge subsides somewhat. By delaying the moment of gratification, you build a reserve of energy that will erupt and shake through your body when you decide to release it.

Slowing down sex and touching your partner all over throughout the process will engage your whole body in the sexual experience. Most of us are used to focusing on our genitals during sex because, of course, that is where the most sensation is happening. However, our skin is a highly sensitive organ that covers our whole body, providing so much more potential for intense pleasure. Why limit your focus to only a tiny fraction of your body when you can feel pleasure throughout all of it?

Slow down your movements, engage your full body, and connect with your partner deeply throughout your sexual experience, and you will be astounded by the new levels of pleasure that you unleash.

Exploring Your Partner

How well do you and your partner really know one another's bodies? Do you know everything that they like and don't like? Do they? How much do you know about what you truly like and don't like? If no one has ever taken the time to touch every part of your body and try every kind of touch, how will you ever have the opportunity to know everything that turns you off or on?

Foreplay is not only for pleasure, but it is also a form of communication. Engaging in extended foreplay is a conversation between you and your partner, a beautiful dance of giving and receiving that we can experience no other way. Sex and foreplay provide us with an unprecedented opportunity to get to know ourselves and our partners in a way that no one else does, deepening our bond in the relationship and elevating that bond to the level of sacred.

Take the time to explore your partner slowly and to allow your partner to explore you. Just as they say, "life is about the journey, rather than the destination," so is sex a beautiful journey of intimacy and sensual pleasure for you, and you are beloved. Be very mindful about the sensations taking place in your own body as your lover touches, teases, kisses, and caresses you. Soak in every moment of pleasure, every tackle, and every chill that shakes your body. Practicing this level of mindfulness can be a deeply meditative process that improves your connection with your body, lowers your stress, and helps to clear your mind of worry and anxiety.

Practice a similar level of mindfulness as you explore your partner's body. Pay attention to every sigh, every moan, every giggle, and every shiver. You will learn your partner's most sensitive areas, which make them squirm with desire and pleasure, and which they would prefer you to stay away from. Gaze deeply into their eyes to connect your souls. Taste their skin beneath your lips. Feel the different textures of their skin. Absorb every beautiful and fleeting detail of these precious moments with your beloved and hold them within your heart and mind. They will be with you always.

Engage in All-Over Foreplay for an Enhanced Sexual Experience

Just as with sex, we often spend foreplay focusing on our genitals, nipples, and other hot spots. As we saw earlier, however, the whole surface of the body holds the potential to experience an incredible amount of pleasure. The rushed and goal-oriented approach to sex that so many of us take compels us to take this narrow focus and neglect the rest of our body. Our drive for instant gratification robs us of our chance to surprise and delight ourselves on increasingly deeper and more exotic levels.

The difference between typical sex and Tantric Sex is often compared to the difference between fast food and a gourmet, multiple-course meal.

The gourmet meal takes longer to prepare, but it is much healthier and ultimately more satisfying and delicious for those who take the time to prepare it. Similarly, slow and sensual sex preceded by long, steamy foreplay is a thousand times more satisfying than rushed sex.

As you and your partner explore one another's bodies, you will naturally find areas that are more pleasurable when stimulated than others. However, it is important to avoid the temptation to focus exclusively on these areas while ignoring the rest of the body.

Kissing your partner's whole body is a beautiful and sensual way to bring pleasure to you both. When you do this, take the time to lick and even gently nibble on different parts of their skin.

You can also tease them with a feather or other object. The light tickle will arouse and delight them as you run it over the different parts of their body, awakening their skin and sending shivers through their body.

A full-body massage is a wonderful way to nurture your partner and help them relax. We hold stress in places we never even realize until they are touched and massaged. Massaging your partner can help them to find these stress points and begin to release their tension, bringing them both sensual delight as well as gentle healing.

Slowing down with sex and foreplay is not only a powerful way to enhance and prolong the sensual experience, but it is also a way to communicate your deep love and care for your partner. When you take things slow, explore one another, and give all-over pleasure, you transform your lovemaking into a deeply intimate and nurturing experience that can bring enormous healing to you as individuals and to the relationship as a whole.

Chapter 20. Sexual Compatibility

One of the most powerful features of a good relationship is sexual compatibility. At first, you could assume it is all about how much you and your partner want the same things in bed. Possibly, how your partner has body features like tits, backsides, dick, or straight shoulders the way you have always wanted. This is not completely off the mark, but sexual compatibility goes way beyond such thinking.

Imagine a relationship where your partner has the exact things you want. The height, the eyeballs, the body fitness, and the smile you always adore, but you cannot understand each other. You cannot tell if they are having a good or bad time. She doesn't know when to let things go with you. He couldn't tell when you are angry, tired, happy, or feigning your emotions too. Do you think you could be a good fit for such a person? Do you think you would relish having sex with him? It is applicable to both men and women. Sometimes, he wants to talk and not have sex, but you have no idea, and you pressed for it. You both had sex, but it definitely won't be one she enjoyed.

Women put on a show sometimes. A woman would frown and scream about everything in the house as if she hated you. But all she wants is you. She wants you to drag her into your arms and kiss her. She wants to melt in your arms and passionately make love with you. If you are sexually compatible, you would fully understand her when she falls into a mood like this, and you know exactly what to do. But if you are not sexually compatible, you might flare up at her weird behaviors. Label her all sorts and storm out of the house in anger.

Men have their styles of attracting you without saying a word too. Each person has a different style of communicating with their partner, and they frantically hope you could understand without waiting for them to explain in words.

Unquestionably, sexual compatibility goes beyond having the same taste in bed. These additional factors can determine how well you would get along in the bedroom and beyond. So, you should recognize them all so you can tell whether if you are compatible with your partner or not yet.

Discover Compatibility

What are the features that you should look out for when you need to determine whether you are compatible with your partner or not?

1. **You both have the same urge for sex:** The urge for sex should be considered paramount in sexual compatibility. Your partner has to have the same definition of sex as you. For instance, "do I consider anal, oral, and so on as sex?" Whatever your answer is, she should have the same answers too. "Do I feel a mad drive for sex at least 5 times a week?" "Can I go up to 5 rounds each time I have sex?" "Is there a sex style, sex position that is so heavenly to me, and does my partner enjoy exploring that same style?" You can begin to relax if your partner has the same answer to these questions; your compatibility level is gaining some scale.

2. **You know exactly what turns her on:** If you and your partner can read each other, you edge closer to sexual compatibility than you can imagine. You can tell when your partner is turned on, and all they need is a powerful fuck till they reach orgasm. You can also tell when you should just give a cuddle and ignore your sexual drive. Your partner can tell the same about you too. You both possess the trick to get your partner up and very hard; you also know things that would instantly turn your partner off. Having this ability is crucial to your sexual compatibility with your partner. If your skills are not convincing in this regard, you probably have a lot to work on. But not to worry, I will take you through how to do it in the coming lines.

3. **Sex environment:** Quite strange but certainly true. We all love to have sex in different conditions. Do you enjoy having sex in a completely dark place? Do you prefer a mildly lit or a very bright room? Or are you the type who loved getting laid in quick, silent places and not even rooms? Is your partner the same? Some people love a man who could slide into the kitchen quietly and turn them off while quinoa or steaks are still on fire. They loved having sex in a quick spot like that, the bathroom, the walkway, the table, and not just the bedroom. You need to find out the position of sex that thrills you more, and then analyze how much your spouse dazzle at such sex styles. It is completely "okay" to prefer having sex in a bedroom, as long as it is how your partners love it too. Otherwise, your sexual compatibility is uncertain.

4. **How much affection can you both display outside?** No hard feelings, but some persons would not even want to hold your hand in public. It is not to say they cannot take your breath away in the bedroom, but the public display isn't just for them. If you are the contrary type, the person who loves to cuddle, hug, and even kiss in public, you might have a rough time getting along with a partner who doesn't fancy that, and it might affect your bedroom relationship. It doesn't get any better when you are both out in a garden or a cinema, and you found couples doing exactly what your partner won't.

5. **How about sex tech? Technology in Sex:** Quite awkward, but it is another factor to consider. Your wife or husband might be electrified by the thoughts of recording your sex now and then. He might want you to share nudes, flirt on texts, et cetera. Your love life would get a zillion times easier if you are the same type too. But if not, it's a complete breakdown that can lead you to a marriage blank.

6. **Is she your crush?** If the sight of your lover is enough to stir something in your spine or your trousers, she is definitely your crush. You are likely going to enjoy every moment of exploration with your lover if you both attract like magnets. Some couples watch porn or bring up another person's memory in their head before they could garner the passion for copulating with their lover; this speaks nothing of sexual compatibility.

7. **You communicate:** Have you ever spoken with a husband who would flatly declare that "my wife would never agree to that" or "this is just what my wife wants"? How does it feel when the wife shows up, and it turns out that the husband was right? Spot on! Couples are expected to be just that. If you are the type who communicate intensely, you can complete whatever your wife was saying. You can correctly guess what she thinks, and you read her eyebrows. You would naturally find it easier to tell when their eyeballs sparkle for sexual exploration. You can tell when they soften at your signs, and you know when they blare green lights on anything. Being compatible in this regard aids sexual compatibility too.

If you can read between the lines and you give it some time, you would be able to establish the level of love and sexual compatibility that you share with your lover. Then, you can decide the areas you need to up your game with him or understand him more when you seem different in a lot of regards. For instance, she wouldn't hug you in public, and she would never have sex in the kitchen or bathroom. What can you do?

You need to ask yourself a couple of questions before making a decision.

1. **Is the difference a big deal?** It is okay to get what you love from your lover. But you would naturally adjust to not getting some. Scroll up and list out the compatibility features your partner does not have and ask yourself if you can let go of them or you flatly can't. You may cross out those that don't seem a "big deal."

2. **Can you adjust?** No doubt, you have other reasons for staying in a relationship beyond sex. However, sex is a crucial reason too. These other reasons may induce you to hang on in the relationship. They could be so strong that you would be willing to pay the price to keep it going, and that would include altering your sexual taste. If you are in a condition like this, then you could alter as much as possible before calling your lover's attention to the areas you cannot adjust to.

3. **Resolved the differences yet?** If you still notice a few incompatibility problems that need to be ironed out after asking yourself questions and taking steps on your answers, then proceed to the following.

Ways to Improve the Couple's Health and Sexual Compatibility

1. **Communicate:** Communication is the key to understanding. You need to talk to each other as much as possible. Share your feelings, thoughts, and ideas. When you decide to share your thoughts on your sexual relationship with your partner, ensure they are in the best mood they could listen to. Perhaps right after sex, before sex, or while at a flirty dinner. Watch their unspoken expression as they weigh your suggestions and be ready to guide them through.

2. **Adjust and make efforts:** You need to understand your partner's tastes too. They have their own ideas and sexual

preferences. They probably don't like the styles you were presenting, or they hadn't given them much thought. Don't put pressure on them. Also, be willing to adjust and switch your taste with theirs. For instance, if your spouse loves sex in a dark place and you want a bright environment, be must be willing to adjust so you can both feel the satisfaction of lovemaking the way you always wanted it. If sex times or the difference in sexual urge is the problem, you still need to talk to them and see how you can both compromises to strike a balance.

3. **Be realistic:** If your partner has a much lower sex drive than you or some differences that are so vast that they cannot be easily overlooked, you need to be realistic with yourself. Do not expect magic and recognize that we have differences that may never be bridged. This way, you can determine whether the circumstances are within what you can stand, or you would walk away.

4. **Get professional help:** If you flawlessly love each other and you realize that the differences are too vast that you can easily fill, it is highly recommended that you get professional help. Talk to a sex or marital counselor. There are always opinions you could use to strike a balance.

With all of these measures in place, you would definitely strike a satisfactory compatibility level with your lover, and you could lead a fulfilled sexual affair. Another entity that can spice your sexual compatibility is romance.

Chapter 21. Making Yourself Attractive to Your Partner

Let's face it. As much as we would like to think that we're enlightened, cultured, and sometimes above surface-level ideas, at our root, at the core, we're all sexual beings who are looking to get off. We crave flesh. We need to cum. And we love the visual appeal of a person that we find attractive. And there's nothing better, or more erotic, than seeing a person that we're in love with all dressed up, cleaned up, and made up. It appeals to all of our senses and plays with our libido. It's the very thing that sets us on a course toward orgasm.

There are several ways that we can make ourselves more attractive to our significant others, and most of these ways deal with tantalizing our basic human senses: touch, taste, sight, smell, and hearing. Those senses are at the center of who we are, and to get your partner and yourself in the mood, and it's best to not just pay attention to one or a few of those senses. Tease all of them!

First, let's talk about possibly the strongest sense that most of us have…

Scent

The scent is one of the strongest senses we have, and as many women can attest, there's nothing that can tease them faster than a man who wears a nice smelling cologne or a woman who knows how to dab on a perfect scent.

Psychologists have, for over a century, documented the importance of the sense of smell. The smell is usually the first sign of danger, whether it's an odd smell in a home or the scent of a fire in the distance. But it can also have a calming, easing effect on us. When our olfactory senses are relaxed, so are we. When those senses are teased, well, so are we. Perfume and cologne makers understand this better than most people. After all, they've built a multi-million-dollar industry that has constantly been growing for century after century. Frankly, not many industries on the planet can lay claim to that.

Perfume making is one of the oldest types of industries in the world. Its roots are older than most established countries, governments, and religions and can be found in scripts and texts from ancient China, India, and Mesopotamia. The world's oldest chemist who delved into the art of making finer scents for wearable purposes was a woman by the name of Tapputi, an overseer of the royal palace of Mesopotamia and a governmental figure of her time. Many of her techniques have been passed down through generations of perfume and cologne makers, and the very basis of what she implemented is still used to this day.

By the medieval period, France and Italy became the leaders in perfume making, and by the Victorian Era, England had become a respected maker as well. Today, many fine cologne and perfume companies, such as Mäurer & Wirtz and Floris of London, have been around for many years and have been long regarded as industry leaders.

You can find a wide variety of scents at many retail outlets, but your best bet in finding great, long-lasting scents is to go to places such as Sephora,

Ulta, or retail giants such as Sachs Fifth Avenue or Macy's. It must be stated up front that, more often than not, a higher-end cologne or perfume will indeed cost a pretty penny. It won't be cheap, and you have to shell out a large amount of cash for Chanel, Dior, Burberry, or John Varvatos. But the good thing is, these scents will last you quite a long time. Cheaper cologne and perfume manufacturers do—for lack of a better term—cut their fragrances with water and other low-end material. The preferred, higher-end scent makers do not. So you are paying for quality, and you're paying a decent amount for it, but you're also purchasing something that's going to last you a good number of months, if not years. With the better fragrances, you only have to use just a little bit for it to last throughout the day. This can result in keeping a bottle of your favorite stuff for many months, if not many years.

So, how do you pick what perfume or cologne to buy? Simple. Plan a day where you and your loved one can head out to one of the stores mentioned above or another perfume vendor and start checking out the scents! Find the ones that you love, that drive you crazy, that put a smile on your face, and try them out. Remember, smell the perfume's scent first before putting it on. There will more than likely be little pieces of cardstock paper that you can spray the fragrance onto.

Do not put on scent after scent. You'll run the risk of tainting the original scent with a new one. You don't want that. Many fine retailers will usually have a small container filled with coffee beans. This acts as an olfactory pallet cleanser. Think of it as a glass of water after drinking a shot of bourbon or a sliver of ginger after eating a few pieces of sushi.

Pick a fragrance, smell it, and then take a hearty whiff of the coffee bean container. When you move on to the next perfume or cologne, your sense of smell will be clean and ready to experience the next one.

Once you've found two or three scents that you're really into, dab a little on your wrists or your neck. If it comes in a spray bottle (which most scents do), spray just a touch of perfume on those areas. You don't want to douse yourself, but you also don't want to run the risk of not putting enough on. Remember, it's not just the scent in the bottle. It's also your natural pheromones. You have to know how both the perfume or cologne and your natural body scent work together. Sometimes what's in a bottle can smell great, but after you put it on and leave it on for a little while, the smell isn't as appealing. And sometimes the reverse is true as well. Sometimes the scent in the bottle might not be exactly what appeals to you, but you put it on, and your significant other tells you that you've never smelled better!

It's trial and error. You just have to hunt down what you like and keep your eyes (and nostrils) open. And don't forget, some people work in those stores who are trained to help you with these kinds of things. Talk with them, and ask them about what their favorite perfumes or colognes are. Have them tell you a little about what they've found to be some of the better, longer-lasting scents. In the end, you'll get a great fragrance, they make a sale, and your partner gets to experience a new you through one of their five senses. It's a win-win-win situation for everyone involved!

Granted, to most guys and some women, the idea of spending several hours in a store checking out row after row and shelf after shelf of bottles of scents may not seem like the best way to spend a morning or afternoon. But remember, this is all about setting yourself and the both of you up for a night (and many nights after that) of passion! So, in the grand scheme of things, a few hours in a store is nothing in comparison to having a thousand-and-one orgasm.

And when we're talking about scent and pleasant smelling additions to our person, we don't just use colognes or perfumes; soaps, deodorants, shampoos, and body washes play a part as well. These items can be a great way to enhance your natural scent and get your partner's senses reeling, and they can interlock with those perfumes and colognes to give a person's body an overall pleasant appeal. A good thing to do is to find the items above that have a similar or adds a complementary scent to the perfume or cologne of your choice. For instance, if a guy chooses to wear cologne that has a scented mixture of tobacco and vanilla, then they should seek out a body wash or soap that has those scents within. If a woman chooses to wear a floral scent perfume, then the body wash should be similar.

And when we're speaking of scent, it's not just what we put on that makes us more attractive to our loved ones. It can be what we do with the room we're in. Scented candles or oils can enhance the eroticism level. A nice smelling home is a great way to get a couple in the mood. Vatsyayana mentions in several passages in the *Kama Sutra* of a "Chamber of Love" or "Love Chamber" (depending on the translation), which is accented to a greater extent by flowers, oils, and incense. Whatever smells you and your partner enjoy, whether it be juniper, citric, lilac, sandalwood, or patchouli, get a couple of candles, oil burners, or incense sticks, and let them fill the room or home.

Sight

It certainly goes without saying (but we'll say it anyway) that a woman in gorgeous lingerie is one of the most erotic, sexy, and beautiful things that a man will ever lay his eyes on. And it's almost an accepted fact that a man who wears a suit somehow becomes much more attractive. These bits of clothing, these things that we drape upon our bodies, they're almost like superhero costumes! We go from a mild-mannered working stiff to a sexy beast just with the simple act of putting on a tie or a little see-through negligee. It's amazing.

Whether it is a power suit, or something from Victoria's Secret, or a little costume you can order online, you should have the initiative to get whatever your partner likes onto your body… and then off your body as quickly as possible if the mood is right!

Before we go any further, let's eradicate one common misconception about men and women. The commonly held myth is that men are way more visual than women when it comes to sexual arousal. While it is true that men probably place visual stimulation at the top of their list (if they were creating such a list in the first place), women are visual as well. The difference is, as many studies have shown over the past number of years, is that men tend to take the visual stimuli and want to act on that desire right away. Women, on the other hand, can take in that stimuli and ruminate on it, let it linger, let it swell up inside their thoughts.

As crass as it might sound, men see a nice pair of legs or breasts, and automatically their brains are hardwired into giving in to almost immediate orgasm. Women see a pair of biceps or a nice butt and want to take a mental snapshot of it and examine it in their heads over and over and over again.

Chapter 22. Spin Your Chakras and Breathe to Ecstasy

There are many practices that you will come across in this book. These practices are fun, and you may find them fascinating! These practices include different sounds, symbols, and sights that will help you on your journey to ecstasy. You will learn a few techniques in this chapter. You will need to practice these techniques in order to perfect them. The most important aspect of Tantric Sex is what you are doing this very second: breathing. It is very important that you breathe properly in order to ensure that you are able to attain the deepest level of intimacy and the highest level of bliss.

Why Is Your Breath Important?

When you breathe right, you are supplying your body with the perfect amount of oxygen. You are also letting your emotions and sensuality flow freely. You will be able to have multiple orgasms and may also be euphoric. Your breath is what helps you last longer during sex. It also helps you ensure that the love between you and your partner is intimate. This sounds like a child's play, does it not? But wait! There is a problem that needs to be addressed. You are holding your breath too much! Every human being does. Focus on how you are breathing at this very second. You are not expanding your chest, are you? Your breathing is shallow. This is not healthy! This section covers three simple techniques that you can use to ensure that you breathe correctly.

Focus on The Source of Your Breath

Have you identified that there is a place in your body where your breathing starts? Do you think it is from your throat or chest, or stomach area? It is not supposed to come from either of those areas. You have to make an effort to ensure that you breathe from deep within your body. To ensure that you breathe properly, you will have to take a deep breath. Take the breath in slowly and trace the place where the breathing stops with your hand. Then exhale. The next time you breathe, you will have to ensure that you take your breath from as low as your genitals. This helps in firing up the energy that you need to have during sex.

Egg to Eagle

This is a great technique to use when you are sitting. You will have to bend into the shape of a ball. When you are bending, you have to exhale swiftly. Bring your hands close to your body and place them on the back of your head. Do you feel your back stretching? Inhale and move up slowly into your sitting position. Stretch your hands as far back as you can. Ensure that your elbows are behind you. You should now feel your chest stretching. Arch your back and throw your chest out. You will now feel all the air rushing into your chest. Continue this exercise. You will be able to breathe well after a few repetitions.

The Wells

The aim of this exercise is to take air into your lungs. You will have to take a lot of air into your lungs. This can only be done when you think of your lungs as wells. You will be able to increase the virtual capacity of your lungs. Keep your arms to your side. After you have inhaled, hold the air for a few seconds and blow all the air out with immense force. It should sound like a gust of wind. Then suck in the air by making as much noise as possible. You will make such a sound while making love to your partner. Through this exercise, you will be able to ensure that the sounds you make during sexual intercourse are intense!

Identify and Worship the God or Goddess Within You

Tantra is the path that most people follow in order to approach God. God leaves you with a divine blessing in every aspect of your life. This aspect also includes sex. You are able to connect with God and the divine feeling only when you are making love with your partner since this is when you are honoring and experiencing each other's divinity. It is believed in Tantra that every man and every woman is a god and a goddess. This implies that you are a divine being and have the ability to attain great levels of wisdom. You only have to be released from your shell. Your self-esteem grows since you are honoring and being honored by your partner. Only when you see the divine aspect of yourself will you be able to see the divinity in others.

Over the course of the chapter, you will be able to identify the divinity in you. You will be able to identify the god and the goddess within yourself and your partner. This is the essence of Tantric Sex. You will also be able to achieve enlightenment. The chapter covers the different gods and goddesses that are popular in the Tantra. You can relate yourself to these goddesses and identify your divinity.

What Is Meant by the Terms "God" and "Goddess"?

As mentioned above, in Tantra, every man and woman is treated like a god or a goddess. This is to ensure that you consider yourself as a god or a goddess and consider your partner as the same. That way, you will honor and respect them in the way you would your god or goddess. You will also be able to honor the power that exists in the universe.

The deities worshipped in Tantric Sex are generally angels or beings filled with light. They are symbols of different energies and relationships. The other terms for god and goddesses are devi and deva, priest and priestess, and daka and dakini. These deities are said to have powers and wisdom in them. This power can also be projected within you. This projection depends on your virtues and qualities.

Goddess is a term that is popularly used in Tantra. It has been used regularly, diminishing its original meaning. It is now used to describe a woman who is in touch with the feminine power that resides within her. The initial meaning stated that a woman who was both nurturing and strong is a goddess. A man is not called god often since god is considered to be a super being according to certain religions. There are some religions and practices that say that a person can become a god or a goddess only when they change some aspect of themselves. But Tantric Sex states that you are a god or a goddess since birth. There is nothing that can be done to change that since you have a certain divinity within yourself.

Tantric Sex states that no matter what the race, religion, or caste of the person, they are a god or a goddess, respectively. By calling a woman a goddess, you are honoring her characteristics of being a lover, hunter, seductress, healer, a wild woman, and a nurturing mother. Only when she accepts these characteristics in herself will she be able to honor herself and be honored by her partner and the people around her. By addressing a man as god, you are honoring his characteristics of being a protector, a provider, and a symbol of power, a healer, and a person with a surrendering nature. He has to accept these characteristics within himself and be honored by his partner! You may display these characteristics, or it may be in you, and you are yet to discover it.

Identify Your Roles and Characteristics

When you begin your journey on the path leading to Tantric Sex, you will have to first identify the gods and goddesses that define you. For this, you will have to identify your characteristics and also identify the roles you play in life. Are you beautiful? Are you a hunter? Are you an entrepreneur? Are you powerful? And so on. You will have to write down all the answers to such questions. To make it simpler, you can create a collage of yourself. You could place your picture in the center of a sheet of paper and indicate all your characteristics and roles through text or pictures.

Once you have read about the different gods and goddesses mentioned in the latter part of the chapter, you could write the names of the deities that you relate to most. For instance, if you had written that you are a hunter, you can relate yourself to "Artemis," and if you had written that you were powerful, you could relate to either "Ares" or "Shiva."

Look Beyond the Superficial Aspect of a Being

Have you heard of the phrase, "never judge a book by its cover"? Everybody has! Yet, we still resort to judging a person by the way they look, dress, or what job they have. You may have made statements like "She is fat" or "He is too short." You may have also looked at the person's bank account before you went on a date with the person or got married to the person. But when it comes to Tantra, there is no such thing as a bank account. You have to look beyond the superficial characteristics of the person and identify the divinity that exists within the person.

There are three essential steps that you have to follow in order to worship the divinity in your partner through the path of Tantra.

You have to first accept the divinity that exists in you.

Embrace and identify the divinity in your partner. You have to establish a balance between the male and female deities. This helps in establishing a balance between the energies in you and your partner.

You have to unite the gods and goddesses within you through the union of you and your partner. This creates the perfect balance between the energies. You can ensure that you will attain the highest level of ecstasy.

Chapter 23. Attainment of Ecstasy

Since you have set the stage and have tried to take your partner on a journey of bliss, it is wise to follow the next natural thing—lovemaking. But we are still in a Tantric moment and ought to follow the way things are done. You still need to follow the ritualistic process to ensure you and your partner enjoy the pleasure that comes with it.

Here, you will enjoy some of those things. But first, you need to understand that bliss is being happy to a state of disbelieve. This is a state where you are in deep delight in such euphoria that supersedes the regular type of joy. It is regarded as the highest form of happiness.

You can only truly enjoy your bliss by being present in the moment. You can also enjoy it when you breathe and channel your energy towards injuring your partner is enjoying every bit of pleasure. It is when you are accepting and giving out love.

This is when you magically activate your body and make the mind still. You channel your sexual energy to get to a higher state of consciousness. The method prescribed here would enable you to get the highest form of delight you will ever want.

Synchronize your energy: Everyone knows that life is stressful. So, you won't always assume you and your partner will forever have a static mood. You must truly understand this before you go into the beauty of this wonderful experience.

Since this knowledge is there for you, the next thing to do is to seek ways to synchronize your energy. If not, it will be only one of you trying to make it work, and that's not what you want at this point. Synchronizing your energy can be done through breathing.

You can check that out. It doesn't matter the position available for your breathing. You also sit with your backs against one another. That way, you are feeling your partner from the back. Ensure you both chants together as you try the breathing synchronization.

Eye gazing: This is one of the essential practices that can't be overlooked, especially as it is the most important you will learn from any Tantra teacher. It helps in getting an intense experience when you are both together and doing everything right.

Looking into your partner's eyes can be very difficult. Looking deeply into their eyes can arouse intimacy, and that's why many people have always run from it. But when you are deliberate about it, you will easily connect better with them on every level. It will make you feel vulnerable, self-conscious, or even embarrassed. These are the normal things you will see by looking into your partner's eyes. The aim primarily is to cause intimacy and openness.

With it, you are going deeper into them. This time, you easily see their eye color, lashes, and expression. You can look into their soul. It might take a deeper breath.

Mix eye gazing with a deep breath: This is something you might find hard to do, but it is worth it for various reasons:

- It helps you still your mind as you focus on a single thing. With this method, your mind is not distracted from what you are doing. Instead, you are kept in the present.

- It emits a feeling of attention. When you stare at your partner while controlling your breath, you make them know you are paying attention to them. This gives off a good feeling.

- You can confront your fear of deep connection. Many are afraid of releasing themselves to their beloved, but with this, you are ready to go deep into the feeling with your partner.

- You can go deep beyond mere prettiness into each other's space. You both will easily overlook distraction.

Pick the left eye: You will need to look predominantly into their left eyes because it receives most of the sexual signals. You have to be as relaxed as possible, and don't be afraid to blink.

If you are ever distracted, you don't have to worry much because you can start all over. After all, it is not a staring competition. Be receptive. Watch out for their body's reaction like squinting, coughing, shifting, and lips tightening. Don't worry. You will eventually become still.

Heart hold: This is when you send signals from your hand to your partner's heart. To do this:

- Place your right over their heart.

- Let your partner do the same.

- Now, imagine sending out love energy into them.

With both of your hands as the channel, imagine receiving more profound love from them.

All that matters is that you are experimenting with different places of your body. Be as slow as you can to feel every energy emitting from your bodies—you and your partner.

Stimulate Their Senses

In Tantric lovemaking, you have to honor every part of their body. In other words, the implication of all this is that every aspect of your body is involved. Thus, for you to create a better connection with your partner, you need to try some of the following:

Mouth and face trace: There are places around your eyes and lips that are so sensitive to touches. You simply have to find them gently. The woman's lip is somehow connected to their genitals, and thus licking or sucking them would give your partner the same sexual feelings they would have usually gotten when you touch their genital.

For them to enjoy it, giving you the pleasure of continuing, press your lips to those of your partner, and make moves. This is not the kissing aspect. Now, use your fingertips to make a motion.

Then, continue to the other area of their mouth and cheeks. You can then blindfold them afterward and give them different morsels, especially strawberries, cherries covered in chocolate, a scoop of ice cream, and so many other things.

Eyes: Let your fingers roam around their eyes because the eyes are the windows to the soul. Be gentle as you touch their eye socket and make circles around the corner, tracing. Explore this part and stare in wonder as you do this.

Nose: This is a Tantric spot that will be useful in taking in the right scent. At this point, they will almost enjoy any scent coming from you. Thus, it is wise to give them something memorable.

Try stimulating their sense of smell by blindfolding them and passing scents, including scented oils, oranges, and wine, under their noses.

Sniff out the different parts of their body like animals would do. Let your nose take the role of your finger in stimulating your partner.

Kisses: As you understand that kisses are of different types. We have the peck on the cheek and the soul-shaking experiencing kiss. With Tantra in play, you are here to stir up their Chakra and also make them release energy from the different parts of their body.

Kissing is one way you can go through every part of your partner's body. You have the chance to use a firm or soft method. Some can even be light or with more pressure in place, while others are shallow kisses or deep ones.

To enjoy your kissing segment, understand the types available.

Lipping: This is the type of kissing that involves being soft on the kiss. It is enjoying the moist side of each other's lips as well as the dry parts. This way, you are connecting on every level.

Tonguing: This technique is such that you use your tongue to lip their lips and touch the inner parts of their cheeks. You can use it to touch the upper palate of their mouth. This is the roof of the mouth. You can even use it to caress their tongues.

Love bite: This should be gentle kisses that should be used to arouse one another. This should be done in a better means than any other.

Suck and blow: These two are together because they are sampling the opposite of one another. It is more like an inhaling and exhaling each other's lips.

When you kiss each other, you should take turns in doing the five steps. It shouldn't be done in quick succession; instead, take as many times as you can. Remember, you have scheduled a lot of time for this.

Hand touch: This is one known for its healing capability. For this to be enjoyed, you might consider massaging them. Take a turn in massaging each other. Start by touching their hands.

Remember their ears too: Don't neglect their ears. Touching or kissing the ear is one erotic thing to do.

Chapter 24. Sexual Intuition

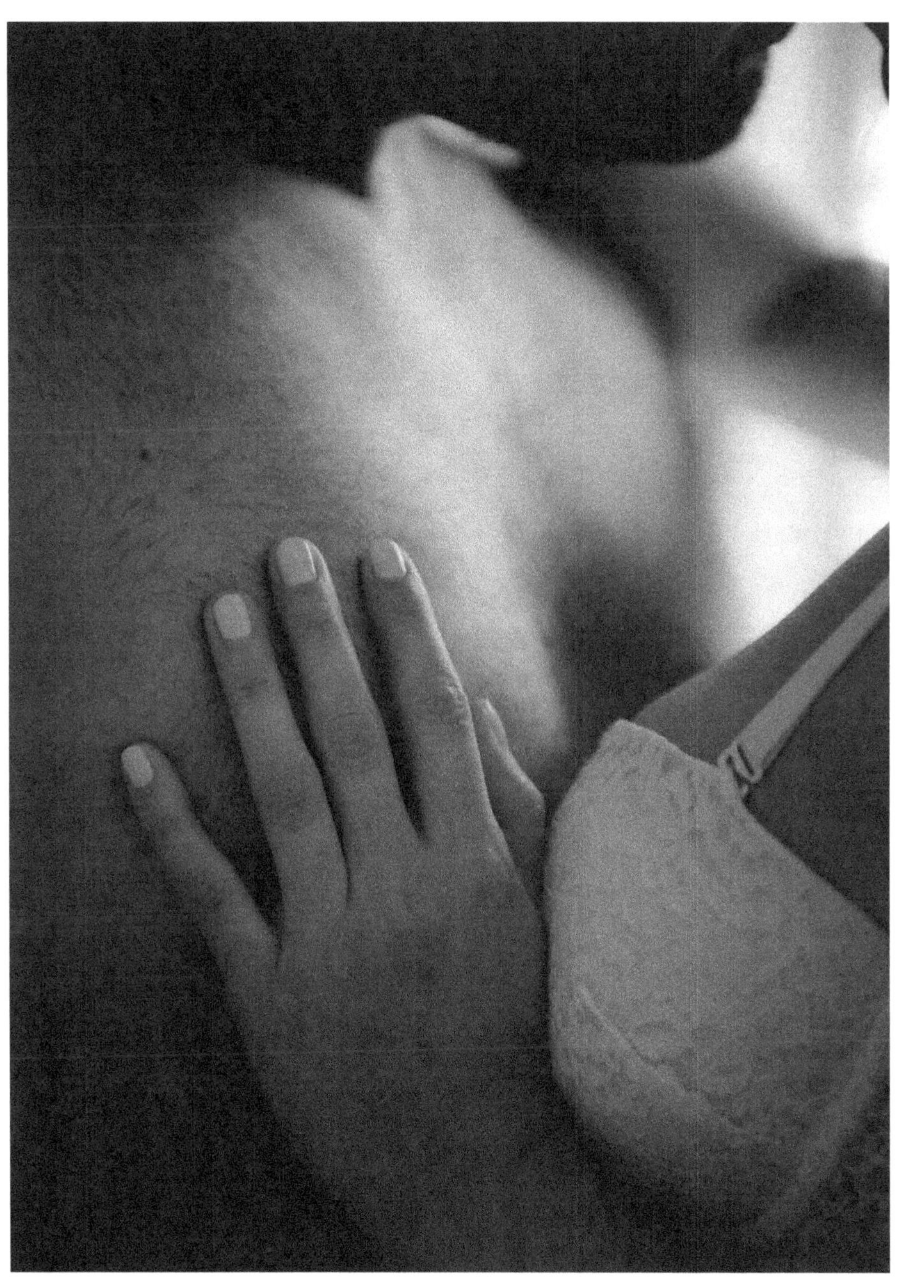

What Is Sexual Intuition

What exactly is sexual intuition? Sexual intuition is somewhat of an abstract concept, and this is because it is something intangible. You can have all the knowledge of sex positions, sex toys, and have lots of experience in bed, but this does not necessarily mean that you possess sexual intuition. Sexual intuition comes from something deeper within.

Sexual intuition can be developed, cultivated, and maintained. It is also something that some people possess naturally. It comes from knowing your body and being in touch with your body on a level that is deeper than just what goes where. It knows your body in terms of being in touch with your desires, your sensations, your needs, and your preferences. It is also knowing and being able to recognize these things in others. Sexual intuition is also being able to adapt to changes at the moment. These changes could be in your own body, your desires, the body and desires of your sexual partner, or it could be changed in your preferences and your desires and the preferences and desires of your partner. It knows how they are receiving you and what you are doing and being able to convey to them what you like and what you want in a sexual sense. Sexual intuition is more than just that, though, as it also knows what to look for in the first place. It knows what to look for in the other person and how to read the answers.

Sexual intuition is all of these things put together. It is more than just knowledge, although that is a piece of it too. It is the ability to look within and at someone else, feel and observe, and adjust accordingly—all of this in a sexual context. Further, it knows that this exists and is something that you want to possess and work on in the first place.

People who do not exhibit sexual intuition may watch porn and become turned on by something that they see on screen, and then enter the bedroom with someone wanting to try exactly what they saw acted out. They have not gone within to see if this is something that they truly desire, if this is something that their body desires, if this is something that will ignite their desires, and if this is something that their partner would enjoy, is enjoying, or even has any interest in.

On the contrary, someone who is sexually intuitive would read about something sexual such as a position or a technique, and determine that this is something real that they would like to try. They then would ask themselves if this is something their body would enjoy the sensations of, if they would like to try this with a partner or alone, and if their partner would have any interest in trying it, or if it would only benefit them alone. They then would approach their sexual partner, and as they began to introduce this new technique or position, they would be able to examine their partner and determine if they are enjoying it or if it is something better left aside.

How to Develop It

To develop sexual intuition, you must put yourself in many different situations and read the situation as best you can. Then, you must communicate verbally. This may seem awkward, but in the beginning, this is the best way to determine your level of sexual intuition. By communicating with your sexual partner something like "I am sensing that you are ready to have sex" or "Am I correct to assume that you are enjoying this?" you will be able to determine if your sexual intuition is correct and if you are reading the situation and the person accurately.

How to Improve It

If you find that you do not exhibit as much sexual intuition as you would like, there are ways to improve this. This also comes down to communication. When you are in a sexual situation, you must ask your partner to communicate with you at every stage so that you can learn to match their feelings and thoughts with what you observe. By doing this for some time, you will be able to eventually match what they are doing or their facial expression to the internal thoughts and feelings that you have learned to match them.

How to Maintain It

Just like anything else in life, maintaining a skill takes practice. The way to maintain your sexual intuition is to practice reading people, especially in sexual situations. This will help you maintain your sexual intuition "muscles."

Chapter 25. For Women and for Men

Specifics on Female Sexual Dominance

The yoni, as I needn't tell most of you, is a very strong organ and incredibly muscular. This effect can be enhanced by the use of Kegel exercises (which we'll discuss in the next chapter). The use of these muscles is key in the exercise of female dominance in sex play. Most indicative of the use of the yoni's incredible strength in the Kama Sutra is the "pair of tongs." This act is achieved by the woman when the man has penetrated the yoni, using her muscles to hold and squeeze the lingam for long periods of time. The pair of tongs may be employed intermittently, so as not to encourage ejaculation. By squeezing and releasing the muscles, the yoni dominates the lingam and the sensations experienced by the man.

The next move is very special, indeed, and probably for my nimbler women readers. While on top of the man, the woman may turn herself in 360-degree revolutions, while the yoni is fully engaged. This is known as the "top" and is not for the faint of heart, needless to say. Do let me know if any of you attempt this one! I'd love to hear how it went!

Those who attempt the "top" will no doubt wear themselves out rather quickly. Should that condition come to pass, women are counseled in Kama Sutra to rest their foreheads against that of their lover and take a breather while the couple is still engaged in sexual union (penetration). At this point of sex play, the man may again take over the more strenuous side of the fun. There's no need to stop when both partners are sharing in the pleasurable workload.

The Kama Sutra advises that women taking the dominant role is the best way for them to fully live out their sexuality. The freedom of guiding the lovemaking and the sense of empowerment is a revelation for many women and should be encouraged by men as the path to greater sexual fulfillment. Due to our respective gender roles, some women have been discouraged from this level of sexual freedom. They deserve it as much as any other woman does, though, and men should welcome it. The woman who is living out the fullest satisfaction of her sexuality is, in essence, showing the man she's with who she really is. Without reservation, she is guiding him to the truth about her desires and providing him with a clear road map, with the route to her pleasure centers marked. This, I'm sure, would be welcomed by almost any man reading. It's said women, in all their complexity and reticence, are too complicated to decipher, but the Rosetta Stone of sex is right there in front of you. That deciphering tool is the woman herself and her empowerment in lovemaking.

Women's dominance, the Kama Sutra advises, should be abstained from by women who are menstruating, those who have recently given birth, and women of material dimensions. As I've said throughout this book, the Kama Sutra was written a very long time ago. While it is, in some respects, quite progressive in its expressed attitudes toward human sexuality, these advisories reflect its age and should be taken in that spirit. You and your partner make all decisions about your sex play, and that includes when and how you will enjoy it. It also includes a fundamental acceptance and love of one another's bodies, of whatever dimensions they are. As partners, these decisions are yours to make, and your bodies are for your personal enjoyment and mutual pleasure. The Kama Sutra, while offering some very useful information and encouragement to couples seeking a more fulfilling sex life, should always be read in its historical context, and this passage is only one of many reasons for that.

The "Work of a Man"

The man's role in sex, for the Kama Sutra, is to provide his woman with pleasure. This pleasure includes the art of teasing her as she teases him in return. The book is clear in its counsel in this respect, calling on men to caress women artfully and mindfully, with an awareness of her erogenous areas and desire to be touched with the greatest possible awareness of her response to those touches. Kama Sutra also ties the "work of a man" to the age and level of sexual experience possessed by their female partners, advising that the breasts are the first area that needs to be attended to in the case of a young partner. In the event of an experienced woman, to whom the man is equal in terms of sexual experience and expertise, the man is advised that no holds are barred.

Kama Sutra is especially clear that every occasion on which partners enjoy each other's bodies should be approached as a new experience. Each session of lovemaking will be different, with both partners participating in the decisions made in the course of their sexual encounter equally, but with women guiding the action and the man responding to her signals. Expressions of passion by the man are part of the woman's pleasure, as these assure her that the sexual bond between her and her man is strong and intense.

The "work of a man" is to bring to the woman the realization of her desires with his body, in every way possible, and to ignite in her the passion she feels for him. He is not there to please himself. He's there to please his woman, with all he does being returned to him by her. This reciprocity, while guided by the woman, is actively pursued by the man in response. This creates between a loving couple the type of give-and-take environment in which sex lives may thrive. Each partner is giving and receiving in equal measure, but the woman engaged in her desires is the birthplace of good sex, in the Kama Sutra's estimation. A woman who is having her needs met will meet those of the man. Thus, it's safe to say that what Kama Sutra teaches is that men need to know which side their bread is buttered on!

Men are also told by Kama Sutra that a woman's eyes will guide him to where she wants to be touched. For this reason, observation is the better part of valor in the love play of a sexually-aware man. His hands follow the signals sent by her eyes, and on them are borne her desires.

Kama Sutra states that men will know they're on the right track when their women's bodies are completely relaxed, her eyes close, and her inhibitions well and truly lost. As love play continues, the man will become increasingly aware that his woman is ready to proceed to intercourse, as these signs are seen. These are common-sense tips about the way most women in bed express their trust in the men they're with. When women feel comfortable, they ready to enjoy their sexuality.

Sometimes, in a hurried world, men fail to read their women and the cues they provide them within the bed. It's extremely important that all men pay close attention to these cues and clues and not assume that their partner is enjoying what they're up to.

Men who are on the wrong track will get some pretty obvious signals from women that this is the case. A sexually unhappy woman can get a little cranky and may go as far as to bite the man (yes, I have heard of this happening and would be very surprised if my readers haven't). Dissatisfaction on the part of the woman may also be expressed by her continuing to urge the man with her body if he climaxes before he should. There is nothing more frustrating than a man who is unable to control his orgasms in order to ensure the pleasure of his partner. Men should be aware that women won't tolerate that for very long. In fact, they will seek more satisfying pastures if men are unable or unwilling to do the "work of a man." The Kama Sutra even gives this option its seal of approval.

The Kama Sutra counsels that, in the event of the woman's continuing ardor, men resort to yoni massage, gently acknowledging the woman's desire by fondling and rubbing her yoni, gently. When ready to continue (when the man has achieved an erection), he should continue with intercourse. Ideally, male orgasm should be delayed as long as possible during any given lovemaking session. We've talked about sexual continence a bit in this book, and later, we'll talk about some exercises to improve control of the traditional orgasm to allow for extended sex play.

Specifics on the "Work of a Man"

Now the Kama Sutra gets a little graphic about what men are to do during the act of intercourse.

On initiation (penetration of the yoni by the lingam), the man enters the woman. In moving his organ forward to enter the yoni, the man is achieving one of the most sublime acts of physical love, in which he is united with his Shakti. By entering the body of his woman with his penis, a man enters the holy of holies, uniting the lingam and yoni in a sacred act of co-creative splendor. This act is not to be taken lightly. The joining of two human bodies in the act of sexual intercourse is a profoundly spiritual one. The lingam enters its rightful shrine, which is the yoni—the gateway to the very heart of creation—the womb.

Once penetration has been achieved, there are several ways of enjoying it counseled by the Kama Sutra. One of these is the act of "churning." The man, taking the root of his lingam in his band," rotates it inside the yoni so that its walls are massaged by the action. This is a mindful act that acknowledges the sacredness of the holy shrine represented by the yoni. The lingam, in massaging the interior walls of this cosmic, fleshly palace, is ministering to it.

Chapter 26. How to Transform Sexual Life and Improve Your Relationship

At some point in your relationship, sex with your partner may become boring or a routine that you just have to follow. If you are currently stuck in a sexual rut with your partner, you are not alone; most couples experience this. If you are stuck in a boring sex routine with your partner, you have got to push the reset button; that is, you have got to bring back the spark in your sex life. According to sex experts, familiarity is the death of sex drive. This is to say that the more you get used to your partner, the less exciting sex becomes. When that happens, you don't have to give up or leave your partner for someone else. The quick tips in this chapter will help to reignite the passion in your sex life.

Some Tips to Transform Your Sexual Life

Liberate Your Body's Energy in a Different Way

Try something new to liberate your body's energy. You can join a dancing class or try yoga. Once you reignite your connection with your body, doing that with your partner won't be difficult. A recent survey found that partners who are sexually inactive felt unattractive to themselves and also experience feelings of sadness. Reignite the spark in your sex life by trying different ways to move and get comfortable in your body.

Create Time to Learn More About Sex

It could be a night. Take one night with your partner to have an uncensored discussion about sex. Talk about what you like and don't like sexually, talk about the hidden fantasies you have, and try new sex positions. If you and your partner have always been doing the missionary sex position, chances are your sex life will become boring. So spice it up by trying new positions. While at it, don't put yourself under pressure; just experiment with sex positions and see what you like. If there are some fantasies you have, and you kept quiet about it out of fear of sounding insensitive, tell your partner "this night." Research shows that men and women have different sexual expectations, and these expectations do not just change overnight. As such, it's important for partners to discuss their likes and dislikes in order to have a pleasurable experience in bed.

Reignite Your Dopamine With a Fresh Experience

Trying something new with your partner promotes bonding and intimacy. Consider activities that might excite you or scare you; it could be an escape room or an amusement park ride. Doing these activities with your partner helps to create dopamine, and, in the process, you get to experience the love and feelings you had when you started the relationship. According to health experts, the brain secretes dopamine and other chemicals, which promotes romantic passion and physical attraction. When you try a new activity with your partner, your brain secretes dopamine, and that helps to spark arousal.

Go on a Sexy Overnight Getaway, if You Are up for It

Go on a sexy overnight getaway with your partner with role play. Decide beforehand the characters you will play, dress up, and enjoy the time with your partner. According to the U.S. Travel Association, couples who go on trips together have better sex lives.

For some couples who are finding it hard to reignite the spark in their sex life, going on a sexy overnight getaway might put too much pressure on them. A better alternative is to spend time together trying nonsexual activities. You can visit a new local spot that just opened around the corner together or go hiking together.

Pleasure Yourself in Front of Your Partner

When you masturbate in front of your partner, they get to see how you enjoy pleasure, and that promotes intimacy. Giving your partner the opportunity to see how you like to be touched and where you like to be touched means you are making yourself vulnerable, and that builds intimacy and closeness. Masturbation benefits the body in a number of ways, and that includes relieving built-up stress, improving our mood, and that is a precursor for more sex.

If you and your partner like adventure, wear a remote control sex toy in front of your partner and let him hold the remote control. This serves as a form of foreplay to get you excited before the main game.

Take a Sex Class and Practice on Weekends

Take a sex class with your partner. Finding a sex class is as easy as setting up a Facebook account. At the set class, you can learn new sex techniques, positions, props, and toys for sex play in a fun learning environment. Don't just learn alone; practice the things you have learned. While at it, don't put yourself or your partner under pressure; take it slow and gradually bring back the spark in your sex life. If you are looking to improve your sexual life and transform your relationship, taking a sex class is a great suggestion.

Have a One-to-One Talk With Your Partner to Air Out Seeded Stress

Communication is extremely important in a relationship, and lack of communication often contributes to dry spells in a relationship. A recent survey found that partners who argue and resolve the conflict were 10 times happier than those who covered the conflict. So if you avoid conflict with your partner rather than talk about it and resolve it, your sex life is heading to the rocks. You'll be shocked that having hard conversations with your partner helps to build intimacy. Don't take offense or be discovered by what your partner says; instead, your goal should be taking measures to improve your relationship. The truth is identifying what's wrong in your relationship will help to improve it. Even if you and your partner do not have the same sexual energy, talk about it, and think of creative ways to fix the inequity.

Get Cozy and Chill With an Erotic Movie

There are a lot of porn clips on the Internet that are couple friendly. For porn websites that offer couple friendly, female-friendly, and queer-friendly clips, sex experts recommend FrolicMe, Crashpadseries, and Sssh. For adventurous and wild couples, sex experts advise attending a weekend sex convention. In the city you live, sex conventions are organized year-round. At the sex convention, you get to attend sex classes and even watch sex play. Learn one or two things and try them when you get home.

If switching up sex positions and techniques and trying the tips discussed doesn't work, you might have to tap into your inner needs. Most people aren't aware that stress and our daily activities greatly affect sexual intimacy. So what you need might just be to tap into your inner needs to get back on track. Do not allow embarrassment or fear stop you from trying new things with your partner. This new technique might make you reach climax and enjoy ecstasy that you haven't enjoyed before. Sex with your partner can feel new and sweet; you just need to push the reset button.

Chapter 27. Use Your Feet to Make Pleasure

The legs are a brilliant case of how gigantic and sentiments of inspiration are discharged. Likewise, while communicating your emotions openly during lovemaking, your legs have a significant impact on the way you hold your partner and what position of lovemaking you can move into. By and by, I don't see the different areas of lovemaking as things one needs to use as a kind of gym of sex. In any case, having a compact body empowers you to permit the assortment of sentiments and urges that emerge in the energy and delight of love.

For example, as a man, it is a wonderful inclination to sit leg over the leg and have my partner sit stripped on my legs eye to eye, with her legs around my midsection. The brilliant blend of weight, warm wet flesh and pubic hair against my private parts, and suspended bosoms against my chest is an arousing feast. Without having the option to sit in that posture, the closest one could find a workable pace be to sit on a stool. In any case, when sitting on a stool, the thighs are not spread open to permit one to love partner to sink profoundly onto one.

Sitting on a seat, the lady who can't let her knees drop sideways can't genuinely open her mystery warmth and fold her legs over her partner.

As of late, a lady companion let me know, "The first run through my present spouse had intercourse with me, he said he had never encountered a lady opening her legs how I can. He continued saying what a heavenly encounter it was. This was because I had rehearsed some leg extends until I could drop my knees sideways."

Opening Your Legs

For a lady, opening your legs can be an incredibly ground-breaking sexual sign and a profound self-contribution. If it is finished with the expertise, it turns into a creative, just as exotic act. Exotic joy emerges for the most part from how flesh contacts and moves against flesh. The joy blooms into bliss when your feelings pass up, feeling warm, open lips against the flesh, and the coal jumps into searing fire. Be that as it may, many delicate snapshots of cherishing erotic nature originate from feeling your partner's skin, weight, and spread of flesh against you in strange manners. What might it feel you want to kiss with lips and privates, but then have your partner's thighs lying against your chest? It's easy if you can twist at the abdomen until your head contacts your legs.

Without endeavoring to be an acrobat in love, though, here are a few different ways to bring more prominent suppleness to your legs.

Synopsis of Sexercise 1—Opening The Legs

Continuously wear a delicate free dress for these exercises, not tight undergarments like leotards. Or, on the other hand, if agreeable, wear nothing by any means, or only a couple of briefs.

The development needs sensible floor space, about the size of a single spread cover. So, remain in such a space where you feel quiet about doing an activity. At that point, place your feet about double shoulder width. If you have tights or socks on and your feet start to slip, take the socks off. It is essential to dodge your feet moving. This could prompt a slight injury.

Hope to check whether your feet are corresponding to one another. If they are spread out, fix them and let the weight load be taken under-edge of each foot outwardly. Try not to secure the knees back an inflexible way. Keep the knees prepared to flex.

Presently let your head hang forward, permitting the storage compartment to follow until your hands contact the floor. If this doesn't exactly happen, take your feet somewhat more extensive. At that point, with hands supporting on the level, gradually dismantle your feet more extensively, keeping up their equal position and taking the weight outwardly of the foot. Continue moving the feet separated until you arrive at where agony starts in the muscles—most likely within the thighs. Bring the feet somewhat together, starting there.

Ensure the hands are on the floor directly under the shoulders. At that point, twist the correct leg at the knee. This will make the left leg stretch by dropping the hips somewhat. Presently fix the privilege and curve the left knee likewise. The subsequent development is one of swinging from left to right. Rehash the development until you believe you have all-around extended within your legs—likely around multiple times toward every path.

At the point when completed, stop in the focal position, inch your feet somewhat increasingly together, take your weight and equalization on your feet, and gradually bring your head and trunk up into the standing position. Rest.

This stretch is to empower you to dismantle the legs more extensively without torment. It applies to people.

The principal targets in extending our legs in a sexercise are to empower the legs to be opened more extensively and for the twisted knees to be equipped for dropping sideways. For instance, of this, the tremendous sexual posture is depicted as the lady lying on her back using her knees twisted and noticeable all around, and the man lying amid her thighs. This implies for the lady that her thighs are still genuinely shut. She needs to drop her knees slanted to let the male lying amid her legs. If the knees can be released further divided, there is a complete opening and solace in the position. It additionally implies different positions are comfortable and pleasant.

Something I have seen is that even if you can do the postures given just sensibly well by and by, during sex, the body is by all accounts experienced differently. One can move into postures effectively and regularly go past what was conceivable by and by without torment. Or on the other hand, if there is torment, it doesn't appear to be taken note of. One's consideration is centered somewhere else.

Another two stretches that guide this are ones that are mainly to broaden the knees falling sideways.

Synopsis of Sexercise 2—The Open Lap

Utilize this stretch in an open space once more, with free apparel.

Sit on the floor and make sure your legs straight out at the front; if it is difficult to sit like this without a tendency to lean in reverse or advances to adjust, put your hands only marginally to the back of your behind. Take your weight on all fours lift your hips off the floor. This lets the heaviness of your trunk dangle from the shoulders and permits the spine to fix.

Twist your knees and bring your feet toward you so the bottoms of the feet are as one and the knees released away from the middle to whatever point they will fall. Utilizing your hands, inch your body gradually toward your feet – still with bottoms of feet together.

Bring your trunk as close to your feet as you can endure while the knees are dropped outwards. At that point, grab hold of the toes of your feet with two hands and keeping in mind that holding them fix your spine. This will likely draw your feet a little closer. In the interim, move your knees downwards towards the floor, enlarging the hole between them.

This is never a comfortable posture for most Europeans, yet there can be a fast improvement if you do the position, in any event, a few times each week and hold for a moment or thereabouts. At the point when you feel comfortable in it, and it gets agreeable, take a stab at keeping the bottoms of the feet together and lying in reverse onto the floor.

Aside from a helpful exercise, this posture is additionally well worth accomplishing for its advantages during labor. It stretches and opens the pelvic region.

Synopsis of Sexercise 3—Foot to Thigh

You need a space sufficiently huge to sit on the floor with your legs loosened up before you.

Bring the correct foot toward the storage compartment, assisting with the hands. Take the impact point of the foot up to the extent that you easily can into the brace while keeping the left leg straight.

Hold the heel well into the prop and check whether you can drop the correct knee down toward the floor. If it is difficult, hold the foot set up with the left hand and tenderly press the knee down with the right.

If the correct knee drops effectively to the floor, take the right foot in two hands and lift it onto the left thigh. If conceivable, the toes ought to be well over to the external edge of the leg. Of course, check whether you can drop the knee toward the floor. Take as much time as is needed. Your body will react if you give it weeks rather than minutes. Step by step, your knees will open, and your muscles adjust.

After holding the position for a moment or so, put the correct foot out on the ground with the leg straight once more. Presently stretch the left foot to the bolster similarly and rehash the technique.

End by sitting with legs crossed before you. If you can, without much of a stretch, do the above time, it might be conceivable to place one foot in the prop—for the man, the heal goes under the balls—and the other heal before it. In any case, put one leg over the other in a comfortable posture—for example, the left heal contacting the correct thigh and its toes under the right calf, and the privilege heal under the left calf.

Chapter 28. How to Maximize Sexual Arousal and Excitement

You can invigorate the sexual hunger and desire both in yourself and your sweetheart by the encompassing you decide for having intercourse, by the environment you make at that spot, by unique activities, and by utilizing extraordinary items focused for this reason.

The Proper Degree of Cleanliness

A few scents can unequivocally stir sexual excitement. This is done in two different ways. Lots of smell receptors in the nose have a direct apprehensive association with focuses in the mind that are dynamic when an individual is sexually stirred. When something triggers these smell receptors, a prompt sexual intrigue and excitement is the outcome.

The body itself secretes substances with suggestive fragrances. Be that as it may, the body additionally produces squanders and emissions that have the contrary impact in a too incredible sum.

The best possible level of washing and cleanliness is, in this way, important to get maximally stirred. The body ought to be cleaned sometime before sex. In any case, an energetic washing and utilization of gigantic measures of cleanser or chemicals can remove energizing real aromas, and a solid smell of cleanser is straightforwardly hostile to suggestive.

Erotic Perfumes or Pheromones

A method for making both yourself and your partner excited is the utilization of suggestive fragrances or pheromone arrangements on your body. These arrangements contain substances, supposed pheromones, that trigger receptors in the nose straightforwardly associated with the mind focus engaged with sexual excitement. They additionally contain substances that trigger sexual energy by their intentionally detected scents.

A portion of these substances give a particularly ladylike imprint, others give an unmistakably manly sign, and others are basic to people. Consequently, arrangements of pheromones are regularly made in uncommon adaptations for people.

Fragrances with the smell of blooms or the like ought to have stayed away from. These kinds of fragrances may smell agreeable; however, they remove the brain from sexual contemplations.

Use of Make-Up and Sexy Clothes

You can energize each other vigorously by utilizing erotic external garments and sexy clothing. You can utilize garments with energizing hues or with hues or shapes, setting off your suggestive dream. The garments ought to stand out for you towards your coziest territories, for instance, by methods for lines or structures pointing that way. Your garments ought to likewise imagine the state of your zones and the state of body parts you find particularly alluring. Your garments should resemble a solicitation to sexual exercises, yet without looking excessively indecent. Keep away from substantial or voluminous garments resembling a weapon. Such garments sign to your partner that you don't need sex, that you fear sex, or are scared of your partner.

Cautious utilization of make-up to reinforce and underline exceptional appealing qualities in your face can build the energy, for instance, some obscuring of your eyebrows or some concealing under your eyes. Overwhelming utilization of make-up will have the contrary impact. It will make your partner wonder what truly is under that make-up, your partner will grope the make as a shield around you, and your partner will be continually scared of upsetting your make-up.

A basic, exquisite, and whimsical, yet at the same time regular looking, beneficiary trim and hair shading can likewise significantly upgrade the energy. In any case, an overwhelming hairdo resembling a significant fine art will remove the consideration from sensual musings and, in this way, have the contrary impact.

A Romantic Atmosphere

A sentimental air will deliver sexual excitement, and numerous fixings together make such an environment. The encompassing must be clean and brilliant. The hues ought to, for the most part, be to some degree discrete and held in a warm tune, however with certain spots having more grounded shading, for instance, a floor covering the couch you sit in and the cloth of the bed where you mean to have intercourse. Having discretely shaded lights out of sight or some beautiful blossoms or fancy items will finish the visual piece of the environment. The temperature of the air must be lovely, to some degree, warm, yet not very warm. Wonderful and loosening up music will finish the image.

Besides, the setting must be to such an extent that you normally drew your consideration towards one another. There should be some agreeable spot where you feel it characteristic of sitting or rests close to one another. The light in the environment ought to be diminished, yet with a to some degree, more grounded light upon where you expect to have intercourse.

Have a Sensual Meal Before You Begin

The nourishment you sometimes eat before sex can significantly upgrade your energy and desire or have the contrary impact, depending on the composition of your feast. You ought to have a feast that animates every one of your faculties. It ought to contain fixings with brilliant hues, and you should utilize arousing and sweet-smelling flavors like cinnamon, ginger, black powder gun, and cardamom. Some measure of solid flavors like cayenne or stew will animate your substantial responses and, along these lines, make you progressively stimulated.

Espresso or tea invigorates the exercises of the focal sensory system, and accordingly, the sexual enthusiasm. A mug or espresso or tea just before the sexual demonstration will frequently improve your sexual state of mind. Limited quantities of liquor will remove pressure and stresses and make room in your psyche for suggestive considerations and sentiments, yet substantial drinking will demolish your sensual goals.

Arousing Videos and Pictures

Taking a gander at pictures in a sensual magazine or at a suggestive video that portrays sexy individuals and sexual circumstances can animate the correct mind-set for having intercourse. The best pictures and recordings are those demonstrating some new and astonishing methods for having intercourse. The best visual material will give you thoughts regarding new things you can do yourselves. Legitimately comic pictures or recordings ought to be dodged because they wakeful different emotions than sexual energy; however, some level of diversion is fine.

The Role of the Foreplay

The foreplay is critical to expanding your energy maximally, and there are numerous things you can incorporate into the foreplay. Kisses and touches are old-style fixings in the foreplay, both when regardless, you have your garments on and later in your exposed state. You should consistently take as much time as is needed to kiss and touch one another, yet you ought to likewise utilize your dream and play with one another in relentlessly new manners.

You can, for instance, tenderly unclothe each other rather than every one of you remove one's garments. Likewise, place your partner or yourself in amazing and fascinating positions. At that point, you stroke each other with delicate developments. Start via touching impartial body regions and step by step, draw nearer to the suggestive zones of the body, and in the long run, invigorate the closest zones by delicate strokes or delicate fingering.

During the foreplay and the sexual demonstration, it is frequently regular that one of you plays a main job, yet you should attempt to move to be the pioneer, either now and then or during various faces in the sexual demonstration.

Sexual Massage

Back rub can be a decent method for improving your sexual energy. The back rub will assist you with relaxing and remove the day by day pressure and stress. At the point when these upsetting components are conciliated, your brain has a more noteworthy spot for suggestive considerations and emotions. The back rub will likewise straightforwardly animate the sentiments and responses in your sexual zones. While kneading, start delicately and increment the force bit by bit. Likewise, approach the coziest zones of your body bit by bit. Be that as it may, you don't need to efficiently. Utilize your dream and do some amazing controls.

Oils and Ointments for Sexual Stimulation

You can discover a lot of oils or balms you can use during sexual back rub that has a stimulating fragrance and a pleasurable consistency. The oils make the fingers float all the more easily against the zones you back rub and increment the joy during the back rub. A portion of these oils is to be utilized on more prominent body parts.

Different oils are particularly made to use in most private body zones. These oils will offer grease to ease intercourse, yet will likewise regularly have fixings that straightforwardly invigorate sentiments and sexual responses, for instance, upgrading the erections of the penis, improving the engorgement of the female lips and clitoris, expanding the vaginal discharges, or making energizing physical emotions by incitement of the nerve endings or arousing bodies.

Chapter 29. Overcoming Anxiety and Insecurity

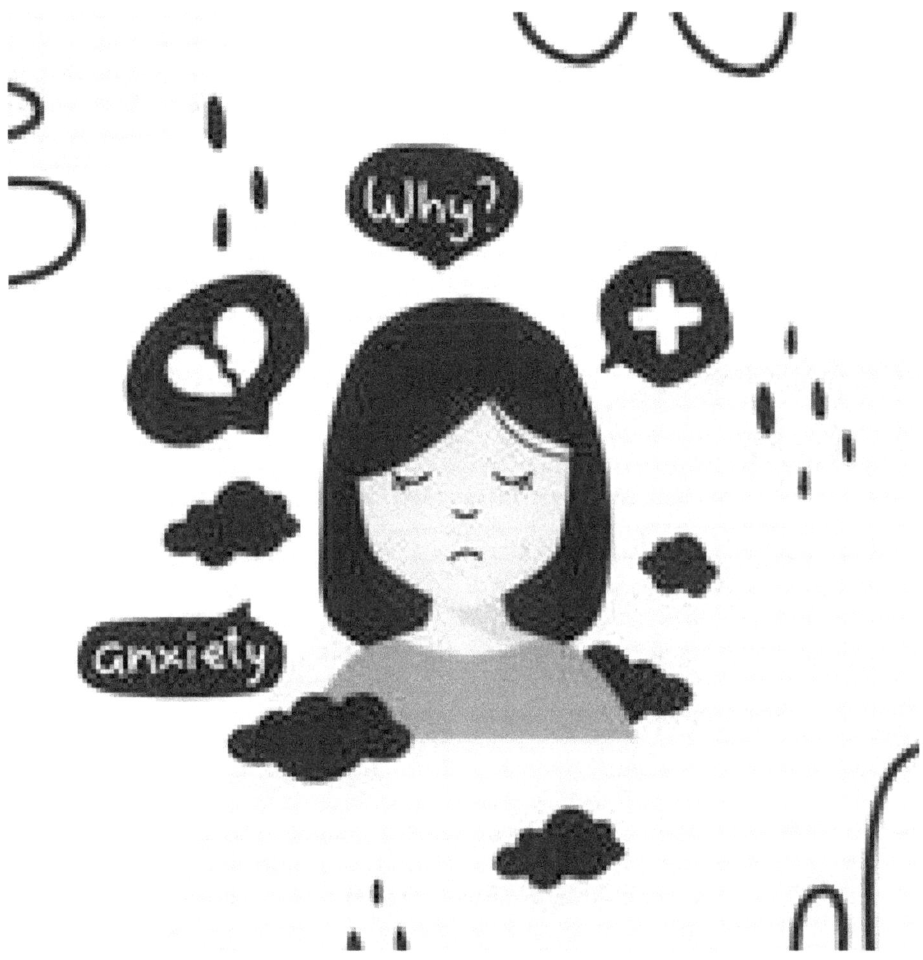

We all worry about several things, most of us lead a hectic lifestyle, and life problems are nearly an everyday occurrence. Most of the time, we deal with our problems on our own, but the bedroom is a different matter. Insecurity and anxiety are two issues that are not going to affect you alone. They will also hurt your partner and instantly kill the intimacy of the moment. You may worry about how you perform in bed, and this actually stops you from performing. Why is that happening? Because worrying keeps you distracted. You are too busy worrying that you will miss out on everything else. You are not focused and present at the moment, and when this happens, you are missing your opportunity to bond and interact with your partner.

Even though this is happening, many people keep worrying about catastrophic results. This keeps happening as if those people are unable to find the switch in their brain and stop. Over time, their worries get worse, and each time, they feel as if they have failed to live up to their partner's expectations. Their mind starts to fill up with negative thoughts that make them wonder if they are as awful as they think and that this is what their partners actually thinks about them. Performance anxiety is a real problem and it happens every time you choose to catastrophize situations that may not even be real. In the bedroom, performance anxiety starts when you start worrying about failing to perform sexually and begin to visualize different disastrous and catastrophic consequences that are going to happen, even though they will probably never happen.

So why do you worry so much? Why do you keep on believing that men should have strong, hard erections that last forever to be considered good in bed? Why do you still believe that a woman is not able to achieve an orgasm with each sexual experience, and for this reason, something must be wrong with her? Where do those expectations stem from? Do you honestly believe that it makes you less of a woman or a man if you fail to meet such expectations? In most cases, people who have sexual performance anxiety are concerned not about their shortcomings but are more concerned about what others will think, which in most cases are their partners. You may be so afraid that your partner will stop being attracted to you or think that you are not as sexy as they thought you were or even that they will find someone else because you have failed to live up to their expectations.

One thing you forget is that we are all human. Something that is supposed to be an intimate, loving, and meaningful moment between two people and helps them connect suddenly becomes something that adds anxiety, stress, and puts pressure on you. This situation keeps getting worse so that instead of growing closer to the one you love, you end up straying from each other. You are human and not a machine. You can think, desire, to have feelings, to sense, and your body does not always do what you believe it will do. Insecurity and anxiety will make you forget everything because your worries will seem larger than what you are doing with your partner in your bedroom.

Nothing else matters, but your worries at that moment and they will eventually grow so big that you will turn away from your sexual encounters. The end of the world has not arrived if a man is not able to keep his erection for long or if a woman is not able to get aroused enough. It is not bad if a man ejaculates prematurely at times or if a woman is not able to reach her orgasm. These things happen. There are times that we all feel stressed and anxious due to the lives we lead. A lot is going on, and we have a lot to deal with, something that results in anxiety being a permanent resident in our leaves that negatively affects every other aspect of our lives if we are unable to control it.

It is a fact that sexual performance anxiety will affect your self-confidence. For instance, would you like someone to see you naked if you feel insecure? The answer, most times, is no, and this will lead to intimacy is the last thing on your mind. It is daunting to seek intercourse when you are feeling insecure, and this is the worst-case scenario when you are getting intimate with a new partner for the first time. Sexual performance anxiety will also diminish your libido even in a non-sexual moment because it will be all that you can think about. There is no such thing as a normal libido, and everyone has different experiences, but when you add insecurity and anxiety to your life, your sex drive will take a huge hit, and you may find it impossible to get aroused.

Anxiety can also cause vaginismus, which can lead to all sorts of symptoms such as sweating, heart palpitations, panic attacks, and various other physical symptoms. A woman dealing with anxiety may have to deal with vaginismus, which is a sexual dysfunction where her pelvic muscles will tighten involuntarily, ultimately stopping her from having sex. A man can have erectile dysfunction. Orgasms in women happen only 57 percent of the time they spend with their partner, while a man's orgasm happens 95 percent of the time. If you are anxious and stressed, it may not happen at all. You may not even enjoy being touched by your partner if your mind is too busy worrying over what they think or how they believe that you are doing.

Performance anxiety is something that happens to everyone: old, rich, young, poor. The symptoms can include:

- Inability to produce vaginal lubes.

- A disturbed state of mind.

- Weak erection.

- Inability to reach orgasm.

- Quick ejaculation.

So what is likely to be the most probable causes of sexual anxiety? Past experiences can lead to such a situation. Many people who are dealing with sexual anxiety had it caused by past experiences. For instance, you may have had sex with someone, and things did not go as you expected. The person may have had slammed you with degrading words about your size or your performance. You could also have had sex with someone, and they complained nonstop during your sex session. You should understand that such experiences are not necessarily going to be repeated with your current partner, and in the end, not all of us can be compatible with every person out there.

Such experiences may have also led you to doubt yourself. Bad past experiences could lead to low self-confidence and low self-esteem. On the other hand, there are times when such situations have nothing to do with your past. You did not have an awful experience, but maybe you have doubts about yourself that led to the uncertainty of performing as well as you'd like for your partner to approve. Keep in mind that your partner may not even judge you by the first few times that you have sex, as they should do. The first few sexual encounters between new couples have to do with discovering and learning more about the preferences of each partner.

There are people who perceive themselves badly, and it has nothing to do with their partner. Sexual performance anxiety has to do with yourself. How you see yourself can affect a lot your chances of developing sexual anxiety. You may think that you don't have the perfect body or that you don't look sexy enough; you may even think that you are ugly. The more negative things you think about yourself, the more you will enhance your sexual nervousness. No person is perfect, not even models. This should not stop you from enjoying one of the most pleasurable experiences with your partner.

Your sexual anxiety can also be developed by the various things that you may have heard. For example, you may have heard people talking about what a standard erection looks like and how an orgasm should happen. You may have heard tales about how long a man should last. Such things are not standard because each person is different, and nowadays, there are many solutions for people who experience sex differently. When you let such tales bother you, you are elevating your chances of being affected by sexual anxiety. You should only think about the various ways you can get better because practice makes perfect.

The first thing you need to do in such situations is to stop being too hard on yourself. There is no need to change anything about you because you are perfect the way you are, and there is no reason to compare yourself to others. Nothing good will come out of worrying. Things will not change for the better but will only get worse. It is normal to occasionally worry, but if you come to the point of dealing with insecurity and anxiety, you will have to talk to your partner so that they can help you. In sex, both partners participate, and you cannot expect to be united if you are on different pages. You should talk to your partner and let them know that you are going through this situation. Help them understand you and let them know that you are working through it as well as the various things they can do to help.

But what can you do to help yourself? You can start by not believing how good you are being based on if you can achieve orgasm or by helping your partner to achieve orgasm. You and your partner are something more than simply orgasms, and you need to respect both of you as human beings. There is no such thing as perfection, and yet life experiences can be beautiful. You should calm your racing thoughts by taking a deep breath and focus on your breathing. Ask yourself why you are worried and if there is a genuine cause for your worries. Maybe your worries are based on assumptions you think are going to happen. Is there any proof for the things that you worry about? If your answer is affirmative, take deep breaths and reassure yourself that everything will be okay. Then, count to five and give yourself time to calm down. Focus on the things that you can control and will improve your sexual experience.

There is no reason for you to worry about being good (or bad) in bed. There is no rating on sexual performance, and the only thing you have managed to do is place unnecessary pressure on yourself when you are the only one trying to rate your own performance. What should matter most is the experience you are going through with your partner right now—the partner you love and care about. Any pleasure you give to your partner is going to be great because you are having sex with the person that you love.

Chapter 30. Aphrodisiac Foods

An aphrodisiac is something that stimulates sexual desire. There are some foods that are believed to stimulate pleasure centers and increase the sex drive and desire of the people eating them. There are different aphrodisiacs in every culture. In the Kama Sutra, the aphrodisiac foods that were recommended included rice mixed with wild honey as well as a mix of ground-up pumpkin seeds, almonds, sugar cane the root of the bamboo that were mixed into milk and honey.

The combinations above may seem a little weird to people today. Below you will find a list of some of the foods that are the typical aphrodisiacs that are used today.

Avocado: This fruit has been considered an aphrodisiac for a long time. The fruit's high levels of vitamin E could be responsible for keeping the spark alive in the bedroom because it was meant to help maintain youth and energy.

Bananas: Bromelain is an enzyme that is found in bananas and is known to trigger testosterone production. The spike in testosterone helps raise arousal in men.

Chili peppers: This bright red spice stimulates endorphins, which can give you the same symptoms that you will feel when you are aroused.

Chocolate: Dark chocolate can give you a chemical spike to make you feel pleasure; this is why chocolate-covered fruit is a common choice of dessert foods for couples.

Coffee: Caffeine is a stimulant that causes more blood to flow through the body. It is also highly thought of to put women into an aroused mood.

Honey: Honey helps to maintain hormone levels while increasing energy.

Olive Oil: The Greeks believed that olive oil made men more virile. It is also a great source of monosaturated and polyunsaturated fats, which are needed to ensure that you are healthy.

Oysters: This is probably the first thing people think of when they think of aphrodisiac foods. Oysters contain amino acids that aid in producing the hormones that are needed for sex.

Pine nuts: Zinc has been proven to be linked to having a healthy sex drive. Pine nuts are high in zinc, which is why they are considered an aphrodisiac.

Pumpkin seeds: These little seeds are incredibly high in magnesium. Magnesium helps to raise the levels of testosterone by ensuring more enters the bloodstream.

Strawberries: This fruit is great to feed to one another as a dessert that will keep the blood flowing to all regions of the body.

Watermelon: This fruit is thought to have a Viagra-like effect on the body because it relaxes blood vessels and, as a result, improves blood flow.

Whipped cream: While there is no scientific reason that whipped cream will boost libido, it can be incredibly erotic to eat with a partner and is sure to put you in the mood.

There are many other foods that are considered aphrodisiacs, such as figs, cherries, pomegranates, artichokes, arugula, and chai tea. With there being so many options, you are sure to be able to put together a light meal or snack for you and your partner to enjoy together.

While it is believed that aphrodisiacs are going to actually increase sexual desire, they have been shared across all races and cultures. In essence, an aphrodisiac is the human's way of wanting to find a way for better sex.

Sadly, the FDA has found that there isn't actually a non-medical approach that is going to work in increasing someone's sexual desire. But, that does not stop people from believing that an aphrodisiac will work.

Foods are one of the most commonly found aphrodisiacs in the world because they so closely resemble a person's genitalia. As mentioned above, there are a lot of different foods that are considered to be aphrodisiacs. Clams and oysters are most commonly associated with aphrodisiacs because of the way that they are shaped and the texture that the present when they are eaten. But, the truth is that they are going to be high in zinc, which is something that many people lack in their diet, and eating them causes a person to be healthier, therefore, increasing their sex drive.

Spicy foods have given some scientific truth to the fact that food can increase one's sex drive. However, this is because of a spice that is found in cayenne pepper known as capsaicin that causes an increase in heart rate as well as metabolism. There may even be some sweating, all of which are going to be similar to symptoms one might experience while they are having sex.

As strange as it sounds, okra is a vegetable that is rich in magnesium but is also a natural relaxant. All of the vitamins that are found in okra are good for your sex organs, which can assist in increasing your sex drive. However, eating okra is not going to increase your sex drive just because you have ingested it.

Herbs are not often thought of as food, but they are used to spice food, so they are still going into your body. One of the herbs that are most commonly associated with love is ginseng, and that is because it resembles a human body. Plus, if you look at the translation of the name, it actually means man root. When ginseng was given to animals, there was an increase in sexual response, but sadly not in humans.

One herb that can be found in India as well as Africa is the Yohimbe, which is thought to have the qualities of an aphrodisiac. It is thought that the Yohimbe will stimulate the nerves that are located in the spine, which can cause an erection without the need to increase sexual excitement. This herb is now known as the herbal form of Viagra. However, if you are going to use this herb, you need to know that there are side effects that can be pretty severe. These side effects are overstimulation, hallucinations, anxiety, weakness, and even the possibility of paralysis.

I do not know about you, but I think I will stick to natural ways instead of risking those effects.

There are plenty of other aphrodisiacs out there that you can use, but as it has been mentioned, science has not actually proven that using these methods is going to increase your sexual desire. But, it never hurts to try, does it? Even though you may try aphrodisiacs, you need to be careful about what some of the side effects could be. Not all of them are going to be severe and permanently harm you. However, an allergic reaction can slow down the desire pretty fast if you do ask me!

No matter what you do, enjoy your lovemaking and have fun getting there!

Chapter 31. Unlocking Intimate Capacity Through Synergy

The best lovemaking experiences come when you and your partner are moving and flowing in harmony with one another. Perhaps you have experienced this for yourself. What is the best sexual experience you've ever had? No matter what "type" of sex you had or with whom, it is likely that you and your partner were embodying the same energy and matching one another's passion. Whether you had rough sex, slow sex, sleepy sex, or spontaneous sex, the best sex comes from a perfect synergy between you and your partner.

The unfortunate thing is that we don't always know how to create this synergy; it just happens. The right environment, the right mood, the right time of day, and some other accidental factors often contribute to our most mind-blowing sex.

The heart of the Tantric Sex practice is learning how to intentionally create the right elements to have the deep, intense, mind-blowing sex that everyone craves. In the last chapter, we learned how to set up one's physical environment to stimulate the senses and nurture deep intimacy. Now we will look at the internal factors that contribute to amazing, long-lasting, and profoundly fulfilling sex.

What Is Energy?

Perhaps the most important aspect of Tantric practice is the energy that you and your partner bring into the experience. Without the right energy, all your setup and foreplay won't be nearly as effective in contributing to the overall Tantric experience. Setup and foreplay can certainly aid you in establishing the best energy for sex, but to get it just right, more intentional energy work is needed. True Tantra is much more about energy than about sex, wherein the focus is on merging the energies within yourself and then merging your united energy with that of your partner.

So, what is energy? Energy is the animating force behind all of the creation. It is what causes the movement of atoms, the formation of matter, and the evolution of life. Beyond the realm of the physical, energy is what composes the soul or spirit. It is what connects us to the center of divine creation itself.

When we talk about our energy, we are in part talking about the electromagnetic field that surrounds all bodies and the electric force within that animates our bodily functions. However, our energy is also composed of the spirit within our bodies, which is also made of energy.

Energy can take different forms. You may hear people talk about "good" and "bad" energy or "positive" and "negative" energy. What they mean by this is that the emotions and intentions of which others "send out" their energy. When someone performs an action with kind and loving intentions, people say that they have "good" energy, whereas when someone does or says something that is fueled by anger or is meant to be hurtful, we say they have "bad" energy.

When we talk about people "sending" energy, we are discussing the actions, emotions, thoughts, and intentions that they manifest. While raw energy is essentially neutral, our thoughts and emotions can "bend" or "tint" our energy to match the tone of those thoughts and emotions. Others can pick up on our energy and interpret our intentions based on what they perceive. Hence, when people say that they will send us "good vibes" or "healing energy," what they mean is that they will have loving and positive thoughts about us and wish us well.

Energy is a complex force that can be used and interpreted in many ways. Since energy is the raw force behind all of creation, we use energy in its purest expression when we create. We often do this unconsciously, allowing our reactive natures to determine what energy we put out into the world. However, when we start to become aware of our own energy and watch our thoughts and actions more carefully, we gain the power to choose the energy that we send into the world, which, in turn, determines what energy we are most likely to receive from others.

How to Recognize Energy

To reach a full understanding of what energy is and how to recognize and control it, you can start to practice in two different ways. First, you will learn how to recognize the electromagnetic field around your own body and that of your partner. From there, you will start to work with recognizing the energy around you as it manifests from others' thoughts, emotions, and intentions.

Learning to recognize your electromagnetic field is very simple, but it will take practice to get good at it. To begin, rub your hands together vigorously. You will start to feel the heat generated between your palms as the friction warms your skin. After a few moments, slowly begin to pull your hands apart, holding them just far enough apart that the skin of your palms is no longer touching. You will continue to feel the heat you generated by rubbing your hands together, as well as a slight tingling sensation.

Slowly begin to pull your hands further apart until they are about a half-inch away from one another. If you can still feel the warm, tingling sensation of your electromagnetic field, then you can move your hands to an inch apart. If you lose the feeling, move your hands closer together and start over.

Continue the exercise by pulling your hands further and further apart. If at any point you lose the tingling sensation, bring them closer together and move slowly apart again. Feel free to start over as many times as you need. The goal is to be able to sense the energy between your hands even when they are a foot apart or more. Advanced energy practitioners learn to shape and move energy for healing, but that is another line of study beyond what we will learn with Tantra.

You can begin to move your energy awareness to the rest of your body with another simple exercise. Bring your attention to one of your forearms, focusing as much as you can on the surface of your skin. When you are fully aware of your forearm, pull your attention to a quarter of an inch above your arm. If you can feel a sensation at that distance, you have found your energy field. If not, return your focus to your skin and begin again.

Like the hand exercise, you will continue to pull your focus farther and farther away from the surface of your skin. If at any point you lose your sense of your electromagnetic field, go back and begin again. Researchers have found that our energy fields extend an average of 10–15 feet beyond our physical bodies, so you can take this practice quite far before you reach the edge of your energy field.

If understanding and sensing our own energy is difficult, learning to sense the energy of others is a much more complex matter. Knowing the energy of the people around us comes from a number of factors. Most of us begin to learn to recognize others' moods and reactions from their body language, tone of voice, and facial expressions at a very young age. This innate sense certainly plays a role in our ability to sense the energy of others, though true energy awareness goes much further than that.

As you grow your awareness of your own energy field, you will slowly begin to feel when other people's energy fields collide with your own. If the sensation is pleasant or neutral, then you know that those people have "positive" or "neutral" energy that is in harmony with your own. If the feeling makes you uncomfortable, then that person likely has "bad" energy.

Another major part of learning to read others' energy is by developing your intuition. We can often tell what others are thinking or feeling in spite of their physical cues, especially our loved ones. We can't always explain these feelings; we just "know." This knowing, otherwise commonly referred to as a "gut feeling," is our intuition.

Accepting and trusting your intuition is the first step in developing it. The easiest way to validate your intuition is to practice with your loved ones. If you feel that you are picking up on emotions beneath the surface when talking to a friend or family member, ask them if anything else is going on. People often acknowledge their true emotions when prompted, even when they feel the need to keep them hidden in general.

You'll encounter plenty of other opportunities to develop your intuition as you go through life. Sometimes you'll have an intuition to drive or walk one way instead of another or to choose one line at the bank or grocery store over the others. Learn to follow these feelings, and great things will very often follow a pleasant conversation, an interesting find, or even the avoidance of some sort of accident. Your intuition is a powerful part of yourself that can aid you in many aspects of life, and it introduces an interesting element in the sexual experience for those who work to develop it.

Using Energy to Deepen Sexual Pleasure

Cultivating an awareness of your energy and your partner's will enable you to harmonize and channel your energies to create a smooth flow through your sexual experience. When both participants focus their intentions on creating a loving, open, and sensual sexual encounter, the results can be astounding.

The first step to synchronizing your energy with your partner is to communicate openly about what kind of experience you both wish to have. If both partners want a different kind of sexual encounter, it is best to compromise so that both feel their needs are met. It is better to speak openly about what you want and what makes you uncomfortable rather than to see your desires collide mid-experience.

When you have agreed upon the type of sexual experience you both want, you and your partner can spend a few minutes setting your mutual intentions at the beginning of your ritual. Including intentions such as, "To have a healthy and nurturing experience together," "To achieve great emotional and sexual healing together," "To give each other the maximum amount of pleasure possible in an open and safe environment," or "To deepen our bond and create an experience that will make us feel closer to one another," are all appropriate intentions.

When establishing the energy for your sexual experience, it is crucial that both partners agree to only engage in sex if it is mutually wanted. Sometimes we get so busy in our lives that we need to schedule our intimacy to fit around our other obligations. However, when the time and day come, we might be too tired or stressed to feel like engaging sexually. Often, an argument or misunderstanding will create tension with our partners, and we might not feel like sex is the best thing to do while there is discomfort between us.

Conclusion

I hope that you have learned a lot about yourself and your sex life and how you can improve your sex life with your partner. It may seem like a lot to take in and process, but as you let this information sink in, it will become clearer to you.

I will provide you with some tips for how you can begin to incorporate this into your life in general as well as your sex life.

The first tip I will share is to begin slowly and deliberately. You do not need to force yourself to begin applying everything into your life, as it will likely overwhelm you and your partner, and this could lead to more stress than anything else. Begin by picking out one or two things that you would like to begin with. For example, Tantric Massage and longer foreplay. These two will go together well, as foreplay is a great time to practice Tantra. You can begin by explaining to your partner what exactly it is, what it entails, and how you want them to support you in this new endeavor. You can then begin by taking the lead and practicing Tantric breathing and massage together. After this, once you are fully in the moment and feeling your pleasure as well as each other's energy, you can keep going with your foreplay for as long as you like.

Remember to remain patient, as it may take some time to become comfortable and familiar with these new practices or techniques. By being patient with yourself and your partner, you will be able to look at the incorporation of these new techniques and practices as a gradual exploration that you are doing together rather than something that must be conquered and mastered in one session.

To solve problems, to strengthening any type of relationship, and to moving past rough spots. Sex is no different, and communication will make your sex life as comfortable and enjoyable as it can possibly be.

By sharing this with your partner, you will be able to communicate about it afterward. This will help to open up a dialogue about sex, which is especially beneficial if you have had a hard time opening a dialogue about this topic in the past. You can discuss the parts you liked, the parts you disliked, and the parts that left you with questions. You can address these together, and this can often lead to a discussion about sex in general. This is the time that you can then ask your partner if they feel like there is anything missing from your sex life, if there is anything they love about it or if there is anything they would like to change. This can also be a time for you to open up about your thoughts and feelings regarding this. This leads to our discussion of emotional intimacy, as this type of communication will lead to a deeper connection between the two of you.

If you enjoyed it, share it with your friends, and they will be thanking you for bettering their relationships and their sex lives for years to come.